Anticipating and Assessing Health Care Technology Volume

Scenario Commission on Future
Health Care Technology

chairman H. David Banta

senior researcher Annetine Gelijns

Anticipating and Assessing Health Care Technology Volume 6

Applications of the new Biotechnology
The Case of Vaccines

A report, commissioned by the
Steering Committee on Future Health Scenarios

1988
Kluwer Academic Publishers
Dordrecht – Boston – London

Distributors

for the United States and Canada: Kluwer Academic Publishers.
101 Philip Drive, Norwell, MA 02061, U.S.A.
For all other countries: Kluwer Academic Publishers Group,
P.O. Box 322, 3300 AH Dordrecht, The Netherlands

Steering Committee
on Future Health Scenarios
P.O. Box 5406
2280 HK Rijswijk
The Netherlands
Telephone: 070-407209

ISBN 0-89838-412-5

Kluwer Academic Publishers. P.O. Box 17, 3300 AA Dordrecht, The Netherlands.

PRINTED IN THE NETHERLANDS.

Foreword

This report, **Applications of the New Biotechnology: The Case of Vaccines**, is the sixth report from the STG Commission on Future Health Care Technology and one of a series of case studies from that project. The STG (Stuurgroep Toekomstscenario's Gezondheidszorg) was established in 1983 as an independent advisory group to the State Secretary for Welfare, Health, and Cultural Affairs (WVC) to assist in long-range health planning efforts. Thus far, STG commissions have examined cardiovascular disease, cancer, aging, and accidents as issues of importance to the health of the Dutch population in the future.

Obviously, health care technology is of great concern to the government. On the one hand, technology is one of the major tools to promote a healthy population. On the other hand, the costs of health care have been rising at an alarming rate in recent years. These two facts, along with the social consequences of certain technologies such as genetic testing, led the STG to establish the Commission on Future Health Care Technology in 1985. The European Office of the World Health Organization (EURO) cosponsored the project. The Health Council (Gezondheidsraad) agreed to cooperate with the project by furnishing space and intellectual and logistical support.

The goal of the Commission's work is to develop sufficient information on future technological developments in health and health care to assist planning for their consequences.

The first report, **Anticipating and Assessing Health Care Technology, General Considerations and Policy Recommendations**, gave the overall context for activities concerning future health care technology. The government and Dutch society as a whole must move rapidly to deal with the consequences of technological change in health care. The first report provided conclusions for achieving this purpose, focusing on the need to develop a national program or system of health care technology assessment.

The second report, **Future Technological Changes**, presented detailed information on anticipated future health care technologies. In the context of STG's studies, this might be considered an 'early warning system' for health care technology.

The third report, **Developments in the Regeneration, Repair and Reorganization of Nervous Tissue**, focused on future applications of neurosciences, especially regarding Alzheimer's disease, Parkinson's disease, and accidents involving nervous system trauma.

The fourth report, **Health Care Applications of Lasers: The Future Treatment of Coronary Artery Disease**, presents a general introduction to lasers in health care, although more detailed information is presented in Volume II. The main purpose of this case study is to examine the possible impacts of one application of lasers: the treatment of coronary artery disease.

The fifth report, **Developments in Genetic Testing**, examines another application of the new biotechnology, the rapidly developing field of genetics. The genetic revolution has now truly begun and it will transform the ways that society deals with its genetic inheritance. The implications of this new technology are far-reaching. The report explores some of these implications and suggests the importance of careful monitoring of this field.

This report, **Applications of the New Biotechnology: The Case of Vaccines**, discusses developments in the new biotechnology. The ability to directly manipulate the genetic structure of organisms has lead to dramatic changes in biological research, and is now beginning to transform practical technology as well. The report presents some of the new developments in diagnostic and therapeutic technologies. The main purpose of the report, however, is to point out the potential applications in vaccine development and possible future impacts of this field on the health of the Netherlands population.

The seventh report, **Computer Assisted Medical Imaging: The Case of Picture Archiving and Communications Systems (PACS)**, presents information on an important new technology. Since the early 1970s, departments of radiology have gradually turned to imaging with computers, and there are now predictions that all medical images, including conventional x-rays, will be computerized. Such a move would have great potential advantages, but the costs to the health care system and society would also be large. It is important for Dutch society to become aware of these developments and to determine the best course of future action.

The final report from the project on future health care technology, **Potentials for Home Care Technology**, gives an overview of present and future developments in an important and often-neglected field of health care. The report also describes and analyses the home care system of the Netherlands, and conlcudes that the home care system is not structured to be receptive to technology. Therefore, the report suggests ways that the home care system could be improved.

As Chairman of the STG, I am delighted to present this report, and I thank the Commission very sincerely for its rapid and excellent work. The government expects to see changes in policies toward health care technology, and I am certain that the report will be a substantial help in that process of change.

The report was prepared by the Commission's staff, which is listed in this report. The staff was led by Dr. David Banta, an American who agreed to spend two years with the STG chairing the Commission. The decision to invite Dr. Banta to the Netherlands was a recognition of the international nature of issues concerning health care technology. I would also like to point out the presence of a Swede, Dr. Henry Danielson, and a Belgian, Professor Jan Blanpain, on the Commission. Dr. Johannes Vang from WHO/EURO was an official observer on the Commission. We are particularly grateful to these outside guests.

The reports have been developed with the help of experts and reviewed by the Commission and by many other individuals and groups representing a wide range of disciplines and perspectives. We are grateful for their many contributions. As with all STG reports, however, the content of the report is the responsibility of the Commission and the STG and does not necessarily represent the position of any of those who assisted or of the Ministry of WVC.

J. van Londen
Chairman, STG

Preface

As noted in the Foreword, this report is one of several volumes resulting from this study of future health care technology.

The purpose of the study, as formulated by the STG, was to analyze future health care technology. Part of the task was to develop an 'early warning system' for health care technology. The primary goal of the project was to develop a list or description of a number of possible and probable future health care technologies, as well as information on their importance. Within the limits of time and money, this has been done. However, given the vast number of possible future health care technologies, complete information on the importance of each area could not be developed in any depth for all technology.

Therefore, four specific technologies were chosen and were prospectively assessed. These future technologies were examined in more depth, looking particularly at their future health and policy implications. Subsequently, the project was extended to September 1987, and two additional technologies were chosen for assessment.

The total output of the project is as follows:

Volume 1. GENERAL CONSIDERATIONS AND POLICY RECOMMENDATIONS

Volume 2. FUTURE TECHNOLOGICAL CHANGES

Volume 3. DEVELOPMENTS IN THE REGENERATION, REPAIR AND REORGANIZATION OF NERVOUS TISSUE

Volume 4. HEALTH CARE APPLICATIONS OF LASERS: THE FUTURE TREATMENT OF CORONARY ARTERY DISEASE

Volume 5. DEVELOPMENTS IN GENETIC TESTING

Volume 6. APPLICATIONS OF THE NEW BIOTECHNOLOGY: The Case of Vaccines

Volume 7. COMPUTER-ASSISTED MEDICAL IMAGING: The Case of Picture Archiving and Communications Systems (PACS)

Volume 8. POTENTIALS FOR HOME CARE TECHNOLOGY

The first report was addressed to an important purpose. The Commission reached the tentative conclusion early in its deliberations that a system for identifying future health care technology would be of limited benefit on its own. The Netherlands does not have an organized system for technology assessment in health care, and therefore information on the benefits, risks, financial costs, and social implications of technology is not available for new or established technology, generally speaking. The Commission saw the need for such a system. Studies aimed at the identification and assessment of future health care technologies must be developed within such a context, the Commission concluded. Therefore, Volume I was developed as an overall policy document, and contains summary material on future technologies.

The second report presented overall information on future health care technology. The report was based on information obtained from surveys done in the United States and in Europe.

The case studies are intended to examine important areas of future (and emerging) health care technology. However, many other potential subjects and applications could be examined. This case study, then, is only an example of what may be possible in evaluating the impacts of future health care technology.

Technological developments in health care are occurring rapidly, and the information on future technologies in these reports will rapidly become out-of-date. The Commission is aware of this fact, and hopes that it will be possible to continue an 'early warning system' that will periodically update such information and assess specific technologies.

This report is primarily addressed to policy makers and to those who are interested in national level policy making. At the same time, the Commission believes that the information in this report is an important basis for future activities in health care technology assessment in Netherlands and in other countries.

Dr. H. David Banta
Chairman
Commission on Future Health Care Technology

Table of Contents

Introduction

Biotechnology is a familiar part of human activity. For centuries plants, animals, and microorganisms have been used to meet human needs. Fermentation technology, as in the production of beer and wine, as well as antibiotics, is an example of a widely used biotechnology. Biotechnological processes are important in the pharmaceutical and chemical industries (119), but also for agriculture and environmental protection. Genetic alteration (primarily by selection) of the plants, animals, and microorganisms used sometimes resulted in new products and/or higher yields. However, no changes could be induced in a specific way to meet pre-defined goals.

These activities have been changed during the past 20 years by implementation of powerful new biotechnological capabilities. These capabilities dramatically increase the ability to manipulate the inherited characteristics of plants, animals, and microorganisms. Ultimately, such activities as agriculture, manufacturing of chemicals, breeding and raising animals for food, mining, and energy development will become more and more dependent on new processes in biotechnology.

The term biotechnology, as used in this report, refers to "any technique that uses living organisms (or parts of organisms) to make or modify products, to improve plants or animals, or to develop micro-organisms for specific uses" (116, p. 3). One well-publicized technique is recombinant DNA technology (rDNA), in which DNA from different organisms is joined to get new characteristics. Another important new biotechnology is the monoclonal antibody, a substance that specifically recognises other structures. Bioprocess capabilities have also greatly expanded during the past decade. Bioprocesses are systems in which complete living cells or their components are used to effect desired physical or chemical changes.

Health care applications of this new biotechnology have come early. Commercial firms began to develop health care applications about a decade ago, and the pharmaceutical industry has become more and more dependent on new processes in developing and manufacturing drugs and biologics. Research and development of vaccines has been particularly affected by these new technologies.

Vaccines are by far the most effective and inexpensive of available methods for prevention and control of communicable diseases. Smallpox no longer exists in the world because the vaccine made it possible to eradicate the disease. In the future, it may be possible to eradicate measles and rabies. Measles, poliomyelitis, diphtheria, pertussis (whooping cough), and other diseases have been brought under control with vaccine use. A number of studies have shown that vaccines are among the most cost-effective interventions in health care, often leading to savings in health care resources. It was for these reasons that the Commission decided to examine the future of vaccine development as influenced by advances in biotechnology.

Using the new biotechnology, new vaccines are already being developed to replace vaccines made by traditional methods, and some vaccines previously not possible have been developed. In the longer run, a number of new approaches to vaccination may be developed. For example, vaccines against upper respiratory infection have not yet been very successful. Research on mucosal immunity could lead to new approaches to vaccines, such as aerosol delivery to promote resistance to these diseases.

In this report, the focus is on biotechnology as a set of techniques that are applied to make products that can then be applied to improve human health. Biotechnology has a more direct human application as well. Direct genetic diagnosis can now be done in human beings, and genetic therapy may also become possible. Human genetic testing is the subject of another case study from the project.

The field of the new biotechnology is very complex, and in some ways is only at a beginning. Although striking advances have already appeared, as work goes on, difficulties are also becoming obvious. Some early - and very optimistic predictions - about future advances have not yet materialized. More fundamental knowledge is clearly needed before certain expected advances can appear. This does not mean that biotechnology does not have great promise for the future. It does mean, though, that the importance of continued support for research in this area must be recognized.

The **organization** of the report is as follows. The first section presents an overview of present and future developments in biotechnology within the health care system. The second section discusses applications of these techniques in the development and production of vaccines. The third section considers consequences of vaccines for health and for society. The fourth section presents material on a few vaccines of particular importance in developed countries such as the Netherlands. The final section contains policy conclusions addressed to all areas of biotechnology discussed in the report, focusing, however, on vaccines.

Section I – Developments in Biotechnology (An Overview)

Introduction

During the past decades, biotechnology has made an ever-increasing contribution to the treatment of many diseases. The discovery of penicillin and a host of newer antibiotics, for example, completely altered the treatment of infectious diseases. The introduction of new biotechnological techniques, including recombinant DNA techniques, expanded the possibilities of biotechnology almost infinitely.

Applications of the new biotechnology in health care have come rapidly. Naturally occurring and genetically engineered microorganisms are employed to manufacture drugs, vaccines, hormones, and enzymes. New tools, such as monoclonal antibodies, will aid diagnosis and possibly therapy. In this Section, a number of developments in biotechnology are discussed that have a great potential for prevention, diagnosis, and cure of diseases, varying from infections and imbalances of the body's chemistry to less well understood diseases including heart disease and cancer.

The actual techniques of the new biotechnology are not described in detail in this report. Excellent descriptions are available elsewhere (54;116;119).

Monoclonal Antibodies (MABs)

Of all the new biotechnologies, those that utilize monoclonal antibodies are likely to have the most rapid and widespread impact on medicine (135).

Antibodies are molecules formed by all higher animals to bind specifically to materials foreign to the body (antigens). They are made by special cells in the spleen, blood, and lymph glands, called B-cells. Once the invader has been tagged by antibodies, the rest of the immune response, the protection against disease, starts to destroy or neutralize the alien substance. It appears that the human immune system can produce tens of millions of different antibodies, corresponding to all antigens that might ever be encountered. Antibodies vary subtly in shape because of variations in the sequence of amino acids used for their construction. Two identically shaped pockets, one at the end of each arm of the molecule, bind to (exactly) matching surfaces on another substance (antigen). It is this characteristic that makes monoclonal antibodies such powerful tools for the detection and treatment of many diseases. For instance, they will soon be commonly employed to detect viruses, bacteria, and other infections, simply by mixing the appropriate antibodies with samples of blood or other body fluids. Other potential applications of monoclonal antibodies include boosting the natural defences of patients; improving the chances of successful organ transplantation; targeting drugs to specific parts of the body; and purification of drugs before administration to patients (135).

Production. Until the production of monoclonal antibodies was made possible through the use of (in-vitro) cell-culture methods, antibodies were obtained by a difficult process of injecting the antigen in a living animal, collecting the serum, and separating the antibodies from it. Disadvantages of this method included that the resulting antibodies were not pure; different antibodies were mixed in the resulting material. The above mentioned new technique uses hybridomas to produce highly specific, homogeneous antibodies. Hybridomas are long-lived cells in culture, produced by fusion of an antibody-forming cell such as a lymphocyte with a tumor cell such as a mouse myeloma cell (86). Through this technique, monoclonal antibodies that are specific for virtually any substance of biological interest can be developed.

Research Applications. Monoclonal antibodies are important research tools. It is anticipated, for example, that by their application a viral etiology can be established for a number of chronic diseases, especially in those cases when the possibility of growing the virus in culture is limited. For example, arthritis and certain chronic neurological diseases might be shown to be caused by viruses.

Diagnosis. The greatest immediate application of monoclonal antibodies is in diagnosis. Because of their specificity, antibodies are already widely used in the laboratory. Monoclonal antibodies are expected to result in improvements in available tests, and in many cases make them easier, quicker, and cheaper to perform (112).

Monoclonal antibodies can be used for several diagnostic applications (173): 1) for assaying hormones, such as female hormones to diagnose pregnancy and ovulation; 2) for diagnosis of infectious diseases, for example, respiratory infections, streptococci, toxoplasmosis and sexually transmitted disease; 3) for cell or tissue identification, as in the diagnosis of cancer or blockages of blood vessels (as with fibrin-specific antibodies). In many cases, the test is simplified.

It may be possible to attach labels such as radioactive isotopes or fluorescent dyes to monoclonal antibodies directed to the surface of specific cells. These could then be injected into a person so that the label would be attached to these specific cells that than could be 'imaged' by one of several techniques. The antibody can also be made against certain hormones or growth factors and could then be attached to receptors on, for instance, tumor cells (44). Alternatively, the antibody could be made against the tumor tissue itself, or against damaged tissue. These techniques might influence diagnosis of such conditions as colon cancer and areas of infarction of the heart by the early 1990s. Specific kinds of tumor and their metastases could be identified in this way. Furthermore, the pathologist might be able to recognize the tissue or the origin of the tumor, and will then be able to predict its growth characteristics.

Simple and rapid diagnostic kits for the direct diagnosis of microbial disease have already been offered by commercial firms. According to advertisements, they are designed for extra-laboratory use or for use in laboratories with no special facilities or expertise. The two main product ranges are a series of latex slide agglutination tests and a range of enzyme immunoassays.

Kits have been developed for diagnosis of AIDS, bacterial meningitis, streptococcus A, Chlamydia, and Candida infection, detection of bacteriuria and pyuria (urinary tract infection), detection of C-reactive protein, toxoplasmosis, syphilis, rota virus, Epstein Barr virus, and Mycoplasma pneumoniae infection. In addition, methods to analyze the immune status for rubella and cytomegalovirus infection can be expected. New developments can be expected in, for example, herpes genitalis.

Future applications may include physician/patient monitoring kits which will allow simple bedside measurement of drug levels. Rapid expansion of the technique is to be expected by the early 1990s, but will take longer for measuring very potent drugs with low blood levels (133).

Increasingly diagnostic kits to be used by the public will become available. At this moment diagnostic kits using monoclonal antibodies already exist for pregnancy testing, ovulation testing, testing for iron deficiency, and testing for acute heart attack (by measuring blood enzymes) (143;173). Tests for sexually transmitted diseases (e.g. gonorrhea in males) and hepatitis may be offered by 1990 or so. Certain screening tests for cancer (e.g. of the uterine cervix and prostate) could be offered by 1995. Other possibilities include skin diseases, peridontal disease, and glaucoma. Kits using monoclonal antibodies for testing of some genetic disorders are also being developed for home use, especially by U.S. companies. Companies plan to develop and market tests for common genetic diseases such as diabetes (72).

Therapy. Monoclonal antibodies also have implications for therapy. For example, monoclonal antibodies are being used experimentally in the therapy of certain conditions such as cancer (138). If and when tumor localization proves practical for diagnosis (see above), it may become possible to extend it to therapy using a higher dose of radioactivity-labelled antibody. This form of radiotherapy would offer an obvious advantage: radioactivity directed specifically to the malignant cells spares the surrounding healthy tissue. Experimental treatment has already been applied to malignant lymphoma, leukemia, and pancreatic cancer, but clinical applications will probably develop slowly.

Monoclonal antibodies simplify monitoring of the blood levels of drugs, such as those against certain bacteria, and thus makes treatment with them more reliable. Monoclonal antibodies may play an important role in immunosuppression in organ transplants and bone marrow purification. These applications are generally either in development or are experimental. Other potential therapeutical applications of monoclonal antibodies in the modulation of the immune system may be found with allergy and auto-immune diseases

The characteristics of monoclonal antibodies make them extremely useful both for development of new types of vaccines (anti-idiotype vaccines), and applications in their production processes (purification of vaccines). In Section 2 and Section 4 some of these applications are briefly discussed.

Implications. The introduction and use of monoclonal antibodies may have important implications for the delivery and organization of health care. Monoclonal antibodies may change methods of screening, and they can improve the specificity of therapeutic measures. In addition to their potential health benefits, therapeutic application may present safety problems. This especially holds when they are produced by experimental laboratories. However, as industry begins to produce more and more of these antibodies, and they are regulated as drugs, their safety is expected to improve.

The largest implications of using monoclonal antibodies can be found in diagnosis. The major advantage of using this type of test in diagnosis is that the results can be obtained in a short time and should be quite precise. Furthermore, their application may result in early rational management of patients, with elimination of unnecessary therapy and diagnostic tests, prevention of hospital infections by specific epidemiologic control measures, and possible shortening of hospitalization. Outside of the hospital sector, general practitioners will obtain access to new diagnostic kits which can be used in their practice. Overall, the quality of patient's care and management may be improved and costs could be lower as a result.

In addition, the number of diagnostic kits to be used by the public is increasing. In many cases a physician will supervise their use, as in the case of diabetes. However, a number of kits will be marketed **directly** to the public. This move will promote autonomy, but it also has dangers. Lay people are not taught to perform tests nor to interpret their results. The ability of members of the public to follow the guidelines of such kits is not fully known, but available information indicates that kits are not particularly accurate in lay hands (38). Furthermore, no test is completely accurate. The implications of false positives and false negatives need to be carefully considered in terms of potential uncalled for anxiety or reassurance, and the subsequent health care consequences.

At this moment regulations for control of quality are lacking. Commercial diagnostic products may be freely marketed in the Netherlands and other European countries, while in the United States the Food and Drug Administration requires that they are subjected to rigorous control testing before they can be marketed. In the Netherlands, industries producing and distributing kits have established a federation, with the goal (among others) of maintaining quality standards. This federation, and industrial companies individually, communicate rather openly with the Dutch government on quality issues. At this moment this may be a satisfactory situation. In future, however, the number of produced and marketed kits will increase considerably. The question of formal regulations for control of quality may, therefore, be an important policy issue in the future.

Genetic Testing

New techniques developed in the research laboratory will enlarge the scope of genetic diagnosis to a wide variety of genetic diseases and susceptibilities. In the long run, perhaps by the year 2000, the entire human genome will be mapped. There are said to be about 10.000 disorders with a strong genetic component. Until now only about 200-300 have been related to specific gene defects. Recombinant DNA technology will make it possible to diagnose directly all 10.000 genetic disorders and will provide probes to diagnose carriers and embryos carrying the disease. The primary technique being used is a DNA probe, in which a molecule, usually a relatively short nucleic acid, is tagged with a tracer substance and is used to locate and identify a specific gene or region of the chromosome consisting of a small number of genes (72). DNA probes are thus extremely specific. The first applications will be for the intrauterine diagnosis of genetic diseases such as cystic fibrosis and Duchenne muscular dystrophy. The approach will then be extended to genetic disorders that become clinically manifest at adult age, such as Huntington's disease.

The main issue with the use of genetic tests concerns future screening. Already, with only a few programs, such as those for the prenatal identification of Down's syndrome (mongolism), this area has been controversial.

At present, genetic screening programs are applied primarily to the fetus and newborn. Diagnostic material is obtained from the fetus by amniocentesis, but chorionic villus sampling is beginning to replace amniocentesis because it can be done earlier in the pregnancy. Improved biopsy and tissue culture techniques for early intra-uterine diagnosis of genetic disorders can be expected. In the longer term, fetal cells can probably be obtained from the mother's blood stream (although such a technique would not obtain amniotic fluid, which contains proteins also useful for diagnosis).

It will become technically feasible in future to test each person for his or her genetic structure, possibly revealing the individual's likelihood to develop certain diseases with a genetic component. Such diseases could include a wide variety of cancers (e.g. breast and colon cancer), cardiovascular disease, diabetes, affective disorders (such as depression), and Alzheimer's disease.

Implications. These developments will lead to a number of complex social and ethical issues. One of the main concerns will be whether screening should be performed if no therapeutic measures are available. The specificity of the tests, and the possibility of inaccurate predictions is also important to consider. Another issue is how individuals can cope psychologically with information on possible future disease. How will genetic screening tests be used in the work place? Finally, how will society react to information on an individuals genetic make-up? Will some individuals be stigmatized? As indicated, the implications, in terms of individual privacy, medical ethics, and the norms and values of society could be profound and far-reaching and therefore need to be analyzed further (72).

The subject of genetic diagnosis and screening is presented in detail in another report from the project.

Pharmaceuticals

Applications of the new biotechnology in the pharmaceutical field promise exciting consequences for medicine and health. The use of new biotechnology is expected to increase the quality and diversity of pharmaceutical products and to improve the methods of pharmaceutical production. The range of products synthesized by recombinant bacteria is often considered to only be limited by demand and economics. In some cases, production of pharmaceutical products by chemical synthesis or tissue extraction methods may be replaced by production from cloned genes. In other cases, applications of recombinant DNA technology may supplant traditional fermentation methods for the production of antibiotics and other pharmaceutical compounds. Perhaps most important, new biotechnology provides means of producing for the first time large amounts of compounds that are otherwise scarce. Thus, new biotechnology may give rise to the discovery and development of entirely new pharmaceutical products.

The pharmaceutical industry is moving rapidly to take advantage of developments in biotechnology (18). The first drug to be produced by the new techniques was somatostatin. The first to be marketed was human insulin for diabetics, partly replacing the animal insulin previously used. In 1985, human growth hormone was put on the market. Genentech, a U.S. biotechnology company, has six other drugs on their way to the market, including interferons, potential anti-cancer drugs, a blood clot dissolver, and Factor VIII, the lack of which causes hemophilia. These new products are more pure or more specific than previous drugs, and often can be produced in larger quantities.

Through biotechnology it is now possible to manufacture natural compounds which can or might cure or relieve disorders which result from imbalances or defects in the body's chemistry, including some inherited diseases. Hormone and enzyme replacement therapy is of use for disorders such as diabetes and hemophilia.

Antibiotics. The production of antibiotics was one of the first applications of biotechnology in health care. Since 1943, when Alexander Fleming discovered the first antibiotic, penicillin, some 100 different antibiotics have become available for human use. A major problem in the use of them, and the major driving force behind the quest for new types, is the resistance bacteria can build against an antibiotic. Resistance to a particular antibiotic can appear in a strain of bacteria in a variety of ways, including the transfer of antibiotic-resistance plasmids from other species or strains (135). The technology of gene insertion is not of direct use in the creation of new antibiotics, since none of the commonest antibiotics are proteins and thus direct products of genes. However, this technology can be used in the modification of existing antibiotics. Through comparatively minor chemical modifications, drugs with different uses can be created. If microorganisms could be used in this transformation, new antibiotics could be created in a cost-effective way.

Another potentially useful route towards the production of new or more antibiotics is through cell fusion. The principles of this technique, which is generally applicable, are quite straightforward. The outer membrane of the cells are stripped away, after which the cells are induced to combine by adding certain viruses or chemicals. Cell fusion creates hybrid or recombinant cells, which contain genetic information from two or more cells. The great advantage is that novel mixes of genetic material not found in nature can be obtained. Pieces of DNA from each of the original cells may swap places. A control region from cell A may displace one from cell B, leading to the expression of a previously dormant (antibiotic) gene in cell B. Through this technique new strains of organisms can be created with unique and, sometimes, useful characteristics.

Hormones. A defect in one of the hormone systems, the systems that coordinate the activities of cells and tissues, can cause serious illnesses. These can sometimes be remedied by supplying the patient with a particular hormone. At present most of the available hormones are obtained from four sources: animals; human organs, blood, or urine; chemical processes; or cell or tissue culture. Disadvantages accompanying these methods include cost, limited supply, and purity. Genetic engineering is likely to prove better than the other techniques for making significant quantities of a variety of substances. For hormones already available, such as insulin, cheaper and better materials might be made through biotechnology. For others, present supply is inadequate to meet demand, as in the case of growth hormone. Other hormones are still of unproven value and larger quantities are needed before their effects can adequately be tested, as in the case of nerve growth factor (see also report from the project on neurosciences).

The gene coding for **human insulin** has already been cloned and expressed in the bacterium E. coli. Human insulin, marketed under the name Humulin^{R}, is the first therapeutic agent produced by means of recombinant-DNA (rDNA) technology to achieve regulatory approval and market introduction (77). The extent to which rDNA-produced human insulin will substitute for animal insulin is uncertain. Human insulin differs only slightly from that extracted from cows or pigs, and incremental benefits have yet to be demonstrated except in some sub-groups of patients. Still, the unlimited supply of the product and its identity to the human protein are important factors in expecting a gradual increase in the use of human insulin over the next years.

The development of **human growth hormone** (hGH) with rDNA methods also illustrates biotechnology's role in the pharmaceutical industry. In addition to performing other functions, hGH is apparently the prime determinant of postnatal growth in humans. Animal GH is available, but only human GH is satisfactory for reversing the deficiencies of hypopituitarism in children. The established market is small, but the drug industry produced it anyway. With adequate supplies, hGH may also be found useful with other conditions including senile osteoporosis, some bleeding ulcers, and healing after burns, wounds, and bone fractures.

Biological response modifiers. Most agents used for immunotherapy were previously known as immunostimulants. Recently, the term 'Biological Response Modifiers' (BRM's) was proposed for the many agents and approaches that can influence the immune response of the host to various diseases. These may include responses to microorganisms, cancer, and immune related diseases such as auto-immunity. The first generations of BRMs consisted of relatively crude bacterial products such as Bacillus Calmette-Guerin (BCG) and Corynebacterium parvum or the antihelmintic drug levamisole. Of these products, BCG has been found to be an effective biological in the treatment of recurrent superficial bladder carcinomas (60). Second generation BRMs such as interferons (IFN), lymphokines such as interleukin-2 (IL_2), and tumornecrosis factor (TNF) are now being produced using recombinant techniques. In addition, monoclonal antibodies (see discussion earlier in this section) can be used as BRM's.

The production of biologicals by DNA-recombinant technology is an important breakthrough, as now large quantities of very pure biologicals are available for clinical studies. In the coming five years recombinant BRM's will be used for immunotherapy of cancer and therapy of various immune defects. Also, monoclonal antibodies will provide better ways to suppress the immune system specifically, temporarily, and reversibly in organ grafting. The production of more purified BRMs with a defined activity, and the administration of BRMs encapsulated in liposomes (added to vaccines) for direct activation of the immune system, will be possible within the next fifteen years.

In Appendix A Biological Response Modifiers, including **interferon, interleukine-2**, **tumor necrosis factor**, and **anti-human thymocyte globulin**, will be discussed.

Lytic agents. Another potentially important development is the use of lytic agents in myocardial infarction (76). The obstruction in myocardial infarction is in the majority of cases (80 percent) due to fibrin-containing thrombi. Such thrombi can be dissolved quickly by administration of lytic compounds resulting in recanalisation, which stops the infarction and reduces the damage. Existing lytic agents are not ideal. Presently available agents are streptokinase (SK) (a bacterial product) and urokinase (UK) (prepared from urine and tissue culture). Both are not specific for thrombi and are associated with systemic side effects and bleeding complications. An additional problem is the high cost, especially of urokinase treatment. New agents in an advanced stage of development are tissue-type plasminogen activators (t-PA), pro-UK and acyl-streptokinase-plasminogen (acyl-SK-PLG). These substances appear to act more specifically, by attaching to blood clots and stimulating other blood components to break down the clot. Their application is presently under evaluation and the commercial availability is expected in the period 1987-1988. In fact, acyl-SK-PLG is already available in the Netherlands. t-PA and pro-UK appear to be better than acyl-SK-PLG and more suitable for application for myocardial infarction. New lytic agents will be prepared by rDNA techniques that are even more thrombus specific, and possibly have a slower liver clearance. This will allow the replacement of intravenous infusion by simpler administration (e.g. by intramuscular injection), thus increasing the possibility of very early intervention of the myocardial infarction. Another possibility would be the use of drugs that increase the endogenous t-PA production for a period of days. Thrombolytic or fibrinolytic therapy may also be advantageous when applied in other conditions: unstable angina pectoris, lung embolism, and venous thrombosis.

This brief overview has only given a few examples to illustrate the potential importance of these processes.

Implications. The new biotechnology has begun to revolutionize the production of pharmaceuticals. It has provided pharmaceutical industry with potent research tools and offers possibilities to further rationalize and economize development and production processes. In the coming decades a number of (natural) substances, as illustrated above, are expected to be marketed. As with other pharmaceuticals, questions of efficacy and safety will need to be addressed. Furthermore, as the new biotechnology products often compete with existing drugs, their relative effectiveness - and relative cost-effectiveness - needs to be analysed (cf. the introduction of human insulin).

Protein Engineering

In protein engineering, natural proteins are modified to improve their characteristics. Information on the relation between the molecule's structure and activity, visualized by computer technology, is used to optimize these characteristics. The structural change can either be achieved by altering the amino-acid sequence by targeted mutagenesis or by coupling the protein to a carrier-molecule.

Knowledge and insight in the structure-activity relation of proteins may result in new vaccines. Information on the three dimensional structure of the surface-proteins and toxins of infectious micro-organisms can be used in vaccine development (see Section 2).

Protein engineering may be of importance for the optimization of the properties of drugs and biosensors. Enzymes or transport-proteins often are of key importance in biosensors. Knowledge of, and subsequent change in, their structure may lead to their improvement.

Applications in Blood Banking

The new techniques of biotechnology are being applied to the production of plasma proteins, such as Factor VIII (lack of which is responsible for hemophilia A) and albumin (168). These are the two principal plasma proteins that are removed from whole blood and produced for special patients (and in many countries, they are sold by the commercial sector). Furthermore, monoclonal antibodies may replace the third principal part of the plasma derivatives market, the immune globulins (115). Within a few years, these new products will probably largely replace natural plasma products. This will have considerable impact on blood transfusion services and the international companies that produce blood components and derivatives.

Gene Therapy

Gene therapy is one of the most radical notions ever put forward in medicine (135). Developments in biotechnology, especially in recombinant-DNA technology, provided the insights and tools for this development. Since inherited metabolic diseases result from absent or faulty genes, the ultimate cure for these diseases would be to provide the patient with the correct genes that enable the body to make the enzymes or other proteins that are lacking and so eliminate the cause of the disease. Gene therapy refers to the insertion, modification, or excision of genetic material to correct a defect (45). The major practical obstacle barring the way to effective gene therapy is that there is, as yet, no sure method of introducing genes into human cells in such a way that they are subjected to the body's normal control systems (135). For the foreseeable future, any gene therapy will probably be of the insertion type. A non-infectious virus, such as a retrovirus, is used to carry particular genes for insertion into defective cells. It will be used particularly in the treatment of diseases in which the normal gene needs to be introduced only in one organ, in which the gene normally is expressed only in cells of a particular tissue, and in which the amount of the product controlled by that gene is not critical. Such diseases include certain blood disorders, such as thalassaemia and sickle cell disease, phenylketonuria, or immune deficiency diseases (21).

This genetic insertion therapy will initially only be applied in **somatic** cells after the person has been shown to have the disease. Use of modifying the genetic inheritance by inserting genetic material into the **germ** cells seems unlikely until far in the future, if ever.

Miscellaneous Biotechnology-related

A variety of other refined and sophisticated technologies may result from progress in this area. One example is the discovery of oncogenes, genes which are associated with cancer formation. They seem to lie dormant until activated, after which they transform the cell into a cancerous form. Their structure is very similar to that of certain viruses, but they are an intrinsic part of the genetic inheritance and not an extraneous infection. If the factors by which oncogenes are roused from their dormant state can be determined, cancer might become preventable. Treatment with so called anti-oncogenes, substances that block the expression of oncogenes, could be another possible development.

Perhaps the most important point to make is that virtually every health-related research laboratory in the world is now using the new biotechnological techniques, leading to the assumption that further progress will become apparent in the years to come.

Section II – New Approaches to Vaccine Development

Introduction

Vaccines are by far the most effective and inexpensive of available methods for prevention and control of communicable diseases (28). A vaccine is a substance that, when introduced into a person, induces the immunity that will protect him or her from an invading organism, such as a virus. Smallpox no longer exists in the world because the vaccine made it possible to eradicate the disease (14). World elimination of measles and rabies are currently being viewed as additional worthy targets (15;50;68). Measles, poliomyelitis, diphtheria, and pertussis (whooping cough) and other diseases have already been brought under control with vaccine use (see Table 1). Although the overall increase in life expectancy in Europe is primarily a result of better standards of nutrition and hygiene, the reduction in the number and size of epidemics of infectious diseases in this century is largely due to vaccinations (129).

Table 1 Comparison of maximal and current morbidity of vaccine-preventable diseases in the United States

Disease	Maximal number of cases	(year)	1983 cases (provisional)	percent change
Diphteria	209.936	1921	5	-100,00
Measles	894.134	1941	1436	- 99,84
Mumps[1]	152.209	1968	3285	- 97,84
Pertussis	265.269	1934	2258	- 99,15
Polyomyelitis (paralytic)	21.269	1952	8	- 99,96
Rubella[2] (congenital syndrome)	20.000 (est.)	1964-1965	20	- 99,20
Tetanus[3]	601	1948	75	- 87,52

Source: Reference 66

[1] first reportable in 1968
[2] first reportable in 1966
[3] first reportable in 1947

In the past decade, developments in biotechnology and modern immunology have opened up exciting possibilities for further progress in the vaccine field. Within the range of future prospects are the development of a number of new vaccines, improvement of existing vaccines and production of, possibly, more inexpensive vaccines (19). New approaches will be of particular value where organisms cannot be cultivated by conventional methods, or where highly pathogenic and contagious organisms are involved so that their cultivation carries a risk to human health. In addition, improvements in existing vaccines can result in fewer side-effects. New vaccines made by traditional methods will probably become available in the near future, such as vaccines for varicella/zoster, herpes genitalis, Hepatitis A and cytomegalovirus (129).

Many new vaccines, such as an improved cholera or a new malaria vaccine, will be most useful in tropical developing countries and may have large effects on the health status of populations of those countries. Of course, their ultimate use in these countries will be determined by a number of factors, not only technological success. (These vaccines will not be discussed further in this report.) In industrialized countries, too, a number of infectious diseases are still prevalent or new infectious diseases, such as AIDS, are emerging. Many of these can possibly be prevented by new vaccines (141).

In the future, it may be possible to develop vaccines against diseases that formerly were, or still are, not considered to be candidates for prevention through immunization.

Some of these new opportunities are the main subject of this report.

Historical Perspective

Vaccines have now been in use for more than 200 years. The idea of immunity to infection is an old one. For example, it has long been known that a person who had one attack of smallpox would not have another (148, pp. 285-288). In India, children were wrapped in clothes that had been worn by those with smallpox to induce a (hopefully) mild form of the disease and subsequent immunity. Edward Jenner believed that infection with the benign cowpox protected against smallpox. He tested this theory in 1796 by vaccinating a boy with cowpox organisms and demonstrating his subsequent immunity to smallpox. Pasteur was perhaps the greatest innovator in vaccines (148, pp. 285-288). He weakened organisms to develop vaccines for chicken cholera, anthrax, and swine fever, and then for rabies. The techniques developed by Pasteur made possible immunization against such common diseases as tetanus (beginning in 1907), pertussis (1914), typhoid (1914) and diphtheria (1926). The isolation of viruses in 1935 and the ability to grow them in culture made possible the development of vaccines for influenza (1945), poliomyelitis (1955), measles (1962) and rubella (German measles) (1969). (Dates given are dates of the introduction of the vaccine in the United States.) (121, pp. 155-156)

The impact of vaccines may be illustrated by the case of smallpox, which was historically the most important communicable disease (65). Smallpox was endemic (occurring in non-epidemic form) throughout most of the world. When it was introduced to America during the Spanish Conquest, its impact was devastating; in Mexico alone, more than 3,5 million people died. In Europe and North America, smallpox persisted until World War II. The last case of the now extinct disease was seen in Somalia in 1977. The total cost of international assistance to developing countries in the worldwide campaign against smallpox was US$112 million (65).

Fudenberg (53) carried out one of the early analyses of the costs and benefits of vaccines, using polio vaccine. He estimated that 154.000 cases of polio were prevented in the United States between 1955 and 1961. Of these, he estimated that 12.500 would have died and 14.300 would have experienced complete disability. The estimated medical care costs for this group of people would have been an estimated US$327 million and the loss of earned income over their lifetime was estimated at US$6,4 billion. He estimated the cost of avoidance - the cost of the vaccine, the cost of administration, the cost of physicians and nurses - to total US$611 million.

This story has been repeated again and again. It is this striking success of vaccines in the past that has raised hopes that the new techniques of biotechnology can lead to further vaccines to protect human health.

Most vaccines at present are a preparation of killed or attenuated (weakened), thus nonvirulent, micro-organisms that are injected into an individual in advance of the person having the disease, with the aim of producing immunity to the disease. The nonvirulent micro-organisms injected carry complicated molecules, called antigens, on their outer coat. Lymphocytes of the recipient's immune system recognize these antigens, which may be proteins, carbohydrates or lipids, as invaders and respond by producing antibodies that bind to the antigens and identify them for destruction by other components of the immune system. In particular, when bound to their target, they cause it to become attached to a receptor present on the surface of white blood cells, which then engulf and destroy the enemy thus branded. Antibodies also serve to alert a soluble killing system carried by the bloodstream and known as complement. Antibodies circulate in the body for a certain time, protecting a person against later exposure to the disease-causing organism. A person then is 'immune' to the disease (121).

There are two main types of lymphocyte, B lymphocytes and T lymphocytes, both formed in the bone marrow. B lymphocytes recognize individual antigens through their specialized surface receptors. T lymphocytes do not always possess this property. B lymphocytes are stimulated by the presence of an antigen, T cell factors, and differentiation factors to divide into numerous plasma cells of identical specificity, which synthesize one specific antibody. 'Helper' T lymphocytes generally need to be present to initiate this proliferation. Other T lymphocytes actually suppress immune responses. Regulation of such responses appears to depend on a balance between 'help' and 'suppression' by T lymphocytes.

Antibodies produced following specific stimulation by exposure to antigen may be any of a range of immunoglobulin (Ig) types. The different classes of immunoglobulins have specific physical and biological properties which determine their function in immunity. Critical to the design of new vaccines is the observation that production of some immunoglobulins requires a local stimulation by an antigenic substance. Parenteral (throughout the body, usually through injection) administration of the same antigen leads to the production of different antibodies, with little effect on mucosal and intestinal infections (166).

Cell-mediated immunity involves several types of specialized T cells. After exposure to a specific antigen, the T cells become activated through clonal selection and proliferation. The thus primed T cells can release lymphokines, which are soluble factors with a variety of defense functions which can increase the destructive efficiency of macrophages and other non-lymphoid cells. Cytotoxic T cells are also capable of directly lysing virus-infected cells (see alsothe section on research needs).

There is often an inverse relationship between the cell-mediated and humoral antibody responses which may be due to regulatory interactions, through suppressor T cells that inhibit the functions of other lymphocytes, as well as to direct blocking of cell-mediated response by antigen-antibody complexes (166).

Vaccines are in common use for many conditions. Vaccines against the childhood diseases of diphtheria, pertussis (whooping cough), measles, German measles (rubella), and mumps are in widespread use, along with the vaccine against poliomyelitis. Tetanus vaccination is almost universal in childhood, and has made that disease almost unknown in Western countries. Adults, especially elderly, are quite often given influenza and pneumococcal vaccines to prevent influenza and pneumonia. Also vaccines are available against a wide variety of tropical diseases such as yellow fever and cholera.

Although vaccines are one of the most significant advances in medicine, the safety of a vaccine cannot be fully ensured. One problem can be that if the pathogen is not killed or attenuated completely, the vaccine itself may be capable of causing disease. Even in their purest form, convential vaccines still contain contaminating materials far exceeding, in mass, the immunologically active ingredients. Such non-essential materials not only cause unpredictable side effects, they may conceivably counteract and neutralize the induction of protective immunity by the effective antigenic determinants. Furthermore, viruses only reproduce in a living system and, thus, are often isolated from the blood of infected animals. There is a chance that cultured cells, eggs, or blood may contain other undetected viruses that can contaminate the vaccine (93). Facilities where pathogens are grown to make a vaccine require strict measures to prevent them from accidental dissemination. Another problem is that some vaccines do not immunize against all various strains of the pathogen. Finally, some vaccines must be kept under refrigeration until they are inoculated, and this can cause problems especially in areas without refrigeration (121). Some of these problems may be solved by applying the new techniques of biotechnology to vaccine development.

Present Production of Vaccines

Most vaccines in present use consist of the organisms that cause the particular disease that the vaccine is intended to prevent (see Table

2). These organisms are killed or otherwise treated to make them nonvirulent, that is, to provoke immunity without causing the disease. An attenuated organism is one whose virulence in human beings has been reduced by mutation in the course of passage through some different animal host, so that the virus becomes adapted to survival in that animal rather than in human beings (93).

Table 2 Important existing vaccines

Period	Technology available	Disease	Viral/ Bacterial	Form
1798-1949	animal tissues	smallpox	viral	attenuated
	embryonated eggs	rabies	viral	killed
	whole bacteria	yellow fever	viral	attenuated
	bacterial toxoids	typhus	bacterial	
		influenza	viral	killed
		cholera	bacterial	killed
		tuberculosis	bacterial	attenuated
		diphtheria	bacterial	toxoid
		pertussis	bacterial	killed
		tetanus	bacterial	toxoid
1950-1980	cell culture	poliomyelitis	viral	killed
		poliomyelitis	viral	attenuated
	polysaccharide subunits	adenovirus	viral	
		measles	viral	attenuated
		mumps	viral	attenuated
		rubella	viral	attenuated
		rabies	(improved)	
		pneumococcal	bacterial	
		meningococcal	bacterial	
1981-1983	subunit virus	hepatitis B	viral	subunits

Source: Reference 66

Vaccines may be made for bacterial, viral, or parasitic diseases. **Bacterial vaccines** are to protect against diseases caused by bacteria, which are small organisms consisting of one cell. Bacterial vaccines are generally prepared from whole bacterial cells. Most bacterial surfaces are composed of lipids (fats) and polysaccharides (complex sugars). Killed preparations of these substances can provoke immunity to the bacterium itself, as in cholera and pertussis vaccine. In the future, live mutant bacteria may be used in producing bacterial vaccines, but up to the present, most bacterial vaccines in use are composed of killed organisms. The cells are killed by chemical or physical treatment. An exception is BCG, which is a live bacterial vaccine.

Another class of **bacterial vaccines** consists of toxoids, in which a treated form of the bacterial toxin, a metabolite, is used as the vaccine, as in diphtheria and tetanus. The toxoid does not prevent the invasion of the organism into the body, but does prevent the disease from developing. This is a form of subunit vaccine. The greatest advantage of a subunit vaccine compared to a killed bacterial vaccine is the elimination of cellular components that do not contribute to the development of a protective response. Some of these components may actually have inherent toxic activity, and thus their elimination is both advantageous and necessary.

Viral vaccines are intended to protect against diseases caused by viruses, such as measles, poliomyelitis, influenza, and mumps. Viruses have a relatively simple and well-understood structure, and their surfaces offer protein targets to which antigens in vaccines can be directed. Viral vaccines can either consist of killed preparations, as in the case of rabies and influenza, or live attenuated organisms, as in the case of measles, yellow fever, rubella, and mumps. Poliomyelitis vaccine is available in either killed or attenuated form.

Parasitic diseases cause a great deal of illness in the world, but generally **parasitic vaccines** have not yet been successful. Parasites are composed of a number of cells and have a complex structure. They are known to provoke immune responses, so it is assumed that with advancing knowledge, immunization against diseases such as malaria and schistosomiasis may be possible.

New Methods of Producing Vaccines

Until the 1980's the number of future vaccines that could be made was thought to be seriously limited. The necessary living organisms or their key antigens were not available for vaccine production or proved unsatisfactory because of the poor levels of protection generated or the presence of side-effects following vaccination. The new biotechnology techniques, monoclonal antibodies, the idiotype network hypothesis, and the concept of the immune response genes, opened up various strategies by which vaccines can be developed (39;95;110). Developments in the clarification of the molecular structure of the cell membrane lead to interesting observations with potentially large implications for vaccine development. Only a limited number of the potentially antigenic sites are important in inducing protective immunity. New technology allows their identification and subsequent production, either by chemical synthesis or by genetic engineering methods. New and future vaccines might include: those produced by genetic engineering and used as standard purified antigens; those inserted into the human host by using vaccinia virus vector (smallpox vaccine); synthetic vaccines, using fragments of synthetic proteins; and new anti-idiotype vaccines (66;95;110;172;174). There is no definable limit to the possibilities for disease control by vaccines as long as relevant epitopes can be defined and effectively presented.

Genetic engineering. With the development of genetic engineering it is possible to concentrate on putting into vaccines only those parts of microorganisms that are essential for inducing immunity. Recombinant DNA (rDNA) technology can be used to produce all or part of a surface protein molecule. The appropriate gene is cloned, and host bacteria, yeast or animal cells are persuaded to synthesize it in large quantities. The antigen product resembles that found naturally in both its physical and biological properties, and can be obtained in reasonable quantities. These so-called **subunit vaccines** will not cause the side-effects associated with killed or attenuated vaccines. For example, by using rDNA techniques, the genes that encode portions of the hepatitis B surface antigen (HBsAG) have been cloned to produce a hepatitis B vaccine (170). In 1986 this new recombinant hepatitis B vaccine was registered in the United States and West-Germany. One of the major problems with the currently licensed r-DNA vaccine against hepatitis B concerns its stability.

Winther and Dougan (166) identify four steps in the development of a genetically engineered subunit vaccine:

1. identification of the protective immunogen on the micro-organism, with the help of monoclonal antibodies;
2. molecular cloning of the gene for the candidate antigen;
3. expression of the antigen in the bacteria E.coli or in other host systems;
4. determination of the immunological activity of the final product and possible enhancement of its immunogenicity.

In the future, rDNA vaccines may be produced for a number of viral diseases, such as polio, measles, influenza types A and B, herpes and Hepatitis A. In the area of parasitic diseases, work toward development of a vaccine for malaria by using methods of genetic engineering is progressing. In the longer run, vaccines against other parasitic diseases, such as toxoplasmosis, can be expected. In the area of bacterial diseases, one example of progress can be found in the research directed at improving the current pertussis (whooping cough) vaccine (56). Pertussis vaccine sometimes has serious side-effects. An acellular vaccine consisting of two major pertussis proteins has been widely used in Japan for the past 3 years and clinical trials of this 'second generation' vaccine are in progress in Sweden. The genes coding for pertussis toxin were cloned in 1986, providing the basis for a recombinant 'third generation' vaccine.

rDNA technology has also been applied to construct harmless live bacterial vaccines (Salmonella, Vibrio) for the prevention of typhoid fever and bacterial diarrhea. The use of rDNA techniques for the development of polysaccharide or (glyco)lipid subunit vaccines is more complicated. In those cases the synthetic approach can become important.

Synthetic vaccines. Synthetic vaccines are a further refinement to the subunit vaccine concept. Research work has demonstrated that only small segments of the antigen need to be exposed to the immune system to provoke a reaction (147). Of these sites, only a few are important in provoking protective immunity, whereas others may frequently induce the opposite effect of suppression which could be detrimental to the host's defence mechanism (95). This observation has increased interest in the possibility of producing synthetic vaccines. These vaccines merely contain peptides (short amino acid chains) or oligosaccharides assembled in the laboratory to mimic a specific site on the surface of a viral or bacterial protein, polysaccharide or glycolipid (147). They should, therefore, be able to elicit antibodies that give rise to immunity against the pathogen (93). The administration of competing and non-essential determinants could be avoided in synthetic vaccines. The first step in developing a synthetic peptide vaccine is to identify the relevant antigen and determine its amino acid sequence or oligosaccharide structure. Monoclonal antibodies are a powerful tool to identify the principal antigenic sites on an organism. Determination of the amino acid sequence is mostly done by deduction from the nucleic acid sequence of the gene encoding the protein. Oligosaccharide antigens are identified by chemical analysis techniques such as nuclear magnetic resonance (NMR) spectroscopy. The synthetic vaccines have the potential of carrying a large diversity of antigens, so they could be especially useful for the development of multivalent vaccines (a vaccine against several organisms).

Synthetic vaccines could be used to make vaccines against antigens of constant regions of the pathogens surface. If such an essential and conserved region is accessible to antibodies, a vaccine that elicits antibodies against it should be a universal vaccine against all its strains (see Section 4). However, the development of synthetic vaccines is still associated with problems. They usually do not provoke a good and lasting immune response and cannot be administered in large quantities (4). In many cases antigenic sites on proteins are dependent on the spatial structure of the protein. Unlike oligosaccharides, it is difficult to mimic this structure with synthetic peptides. A synthetic peptide, unlike an attenuated virus, does not replicate, and so substances called adjuvants must be added to the vaccine to increase the level and duration of immunity. For synthetic vaccines to be effective, the choice of the proper carrier and adjuvant is important. It seems likely that synthetic vaccines will be particularly useful for organisms/strains that, for instance, grow poorly in cell culture, are very unstable, or show poor immunization rates (11). This seems especially the case if the antigens involved are polysaccharides or glycolipids, since these antigens cannot be easily obtained through rDNA technology.

Studies using synthetic peptides have been reported for a number of diseases, including pneumonia, diphtheria, cholera, influenza, and hepatitis B (42;93). However, none of them has yet reached the stage of clinical trial. In spite of rapid progress in the past few years, synthetic vaccines are still at their early developmental stage (95).

Viral (and other) vectors. Another approach receiving increased attention is that of using viral vectors as a means of carrying antigens with the aim of vaccination. Paoletti and Moss began to investigate the use of vaccinia recombinants in 1982 (10;125). Research is based on the idea that the live virus, e.g. vaccinia, will express a foreign gene inserted into its DNA when it is applied to an animal; this will subsequently lead to an immune response to the product of this foreign gene. Protection has already been demonstrated in animals with vaccinia as a vector for a number of diseases, such as hepatitis B, herpes simplex virus type 1, influenza,and rabies (12). Its proved efficacy, stability, broad applicability, stimulation of both cell-mediated and humoral antibody responses, low cost, and ease of administration, together with the possibility of including in it multiple foreign genes, make vaccinia an outstanding model of a vaccine vector for a range of important diseases (108;109;151). However, the use of vaccinia as a vector has certain drawbacks, such as the still high level of immunity to this virus in the community and potential side effects of the vaccination. Severe, sometimes fatal, reactions occur at the rate of 1 or 2 per million vaccinations (12). There is need to be certain that the introduction of new genes does not transfer virulence factors, tumor promoting activity, or other undesirable properties from the donor pathogen to the vector (109).

The use of other carriers such as adenovirus, herpesvirus, and attenuated Salmonella strains are being investigated as possible alternatives, especially for use against diseases of the respiratory tract and enteric (intestinal) diseases (134). It is possible that these relatively safe enteric bacteria may serve as effective carriers of oral vaccines for other pathogens, the defence against which necessitates the induction of mucosal and systemic immunity (95). Furthermore, the oral route would be ideal for mass vaccination. However, with a few exceptions, until now this route has been the least effective. Few vaccines possess the absorption properties or can withstand the hostile environment of the gastrointestinal tract. Attenuated mycobacteria, with their adjuvant properties for both T-cell mediated and humoral immunity, are also possible vectors, provided the genetic engineering problems can be solved.

Anti-idiotype antibodies. One of the newest approaches in vaccine development is the use of anti-idiotype antibodies. Anti-idiotype antibodies are antibodies of which the variable part possesses antigenic determinants (idiotopes) that are closely related to the epitopes on the original antigen (110). They form an 'internal image' of the antigen which is recognized by the idiotype antibody. Because of this characteristic, they can act similarly to the antigen in the stimulation of antibody production. In the immune system, a network of idiotypes, anti-idiotypes, and anti-anti-idiotypes regulate the immune response. Disorders of such networks may underlie autoimmune diseases such as rheumatoid arthritis and myasthenia gravis.

The specificity of anti-idiotype antibodies is interesting for vaccine development. Unlike an attenuated infectious agent, which may carry other antigenetic determinants besides the one that induces protective immunity, an anti-idiotype triggers an antibody response only to the one antigenic determinant whose internal image it bears. Anti-idiotype vaccines may be used in the future in case the antigen used to stimulate the idiotype is difficult to obtain, when it is toxic, or even when it is non-immunogenic. The antigenic parts of many bacteria and protozoa consist of carbohydrates and fats and cannot be made by recombinant methods or synthetically. These vaccines could be particularly effective in the case of infectious organisms coated with polysaccharide capsules, to which infants cannot respond immunologically until the age of approximately 2 years (80). An anti-idiotype vaccine could mimic the structure of this envelope material, but because the anti-idiotype is a protein, it would elicit an immune response. All three leading causes of bacterial meningitis in infants - Hemophilus influenzae, Streptococcus pneumoniae, and Neisseria meningitidis - have polysaccharide capsules, which presumably can be mimicked by anti-idiotypes.

Immunization with anti-idiotype antibodies has been successful in inducing specific responses to a wide spectrum of foreign antigens, including parasites, bacteria, viruses,and tumors.

Several factors could limit the use of anti-idiotypes as human vaccines. The use of an anti-idiotype serum made in other animals could cause fever and allergic reactions in some people. The inherent uniqueness of anti-idiotype vaccines could make them potentially impractical to be applied to the diverse human population (95). Because of the complexity of the idiotype network, the effect of an anti-idiotype may not always be protective. Though many anti-idiotypes appear to respond similarly to the antigen itself, others may exert suppressive effects on the immune system (80).

In the future, anti-idiotypes may prove effective against cancer, both as a vaccine and a treatment. Administration of a monoclonal antibody to an antigenic determinant on the surface of the cancer cells may induce the production of the anti-idiotype of the antibody. The anti-idiotype carries an internal image of the cancer antigen. Injection of the anti-idiotype causes the production of an antibody that could react with the tumor antigen.

Improving Antigenicity of Vaccines - Adjuvants

In the development of rDNA and synthetic vaccines not only the sequence of the aminoacids, but also their configuration (spatial conformation) and molecular size plays a role in eliciting immune response. If the immunogenic activity in animals of experimental vaccination is low, the peptide or protein may require special carriers or adjuvants to encourage it to fold in the proper conformation and thus to mimic its original shape. Better knowledge of how antigens are presented would help in the choice of carrier molecules and adjuvants to be used with future vaccines. Advances in protein engineering may thus be important in vaccine development in the future. The synthesis of oligopeptides has been simplified and computer programs facilitate the plotting of the three-dimensional structure of proteins, so that the location and presentation of important antigenic determinants, epitopes, can be predicted (33;109).

Adjuvants are a diverse collection of materials to stimulate and increase the duration of the immune response, and thus assist in a correct presentation of the antigen. Aluminum hydroxide is often used as an adjuvant in human vaccines, and is applicable to subunit and synthetic peptide vaccines. The antigen is adsorbed onto the aluminum hydroxide particles and is released slowly after injection.

Recent research has discovered potentially new adjuvants, such as micelles, liposomes, and iscoms (immunostimulating complexes). Aggregation of the peptide into clumps (micelles) or incorporation in phospholipids (liposomes) gives a substantial immunological enhancement (42;66;149). In an iscom, protective immunity stimulating envelope proteins (peplomers) are attached to the micelle form of a glucoside. Antibody titers (concentration) induced by this technique are up to ten times higher than with whole cell vaccination (103). Muramyl dipeptide (MDP), a synthetic derivate of the active site of the cell membrane of mycobacteria, is an immunostimulant which significantly increases the immune response of diphteria-toxin peptides when linked to it as a carrier-adjuvant.

More research is essential to obtain an adequate immune responce for every type of antigen.

Research Needs

Although vaccines are clearly improving, immunity against mucosal infections (respiratory, genital, and enteral infections) is difficult to produce. For example, vaccines against upper respiratory infection such as parainfluenza in children have not been very successful. In contrast, vaccines against systemic infectious diseases and toxin producing infections provide excellent immunity.

Mucosal immunity depends on the common mucosal immune system which functions more or less independently of the immunologic functions in the body as a whole and in the blood stream. To obtain optimal mucosal immunity, methods of vaccination may be required that are different from those used for induction of systemic immunity (for example, place and method of administration, live versus inactivated vaccine, use of vector). Further knowledge of mucosal immune mechanisms and ways of stimulating these mechanisms of the immune system are needed. Recombinant DNA technology may be a particular useful tool to obtain this knowledge. Bacteria which can achieve limited penetration of the intestinal mucosa after oral administration hold the promise of stimulating IgA antibodies and of inducing effective immunity at the mucosal surface, which is difficult to achieve if non-living vaccines are used (33;109).

Biotechnology has furnished new research tools for developing knowledge concerning parasites and the diseases that they cause. Without such knowledge, as indicated above, vaccines will not be possible in this area.

The immune system is complex and not yet fully understood. Apparently both cellular and humoral reactions can be involved in the immune response. An ideal vaccine should induce memory for both humoral and cell-mediated effectors of immunity. Increased understanding of the mechanisms involved may lead to different and/or improved approaches in the prophylaxis or treatment of infections. For blood borne diseases, humoral immunity would be important for both the prevention of infection at the site of entry and the subsequent clearance of the pathogen and thus recovery from the disease. Cell-mediated immunological processes, acting alone or in conjunction with specific antibodies, may contribute to protective immunity and potentially to immunopathological processes. Antigens which do not induce neutralizing antibodies yet activate helper T cells for subsequent enhancement of protective humoral response upon infection could be as effective as those provoking initial neutralizing antibodies. If molecules could be designed able to selectively stimulate helper T cells, vaccine development would benefit (101). Antibody-dependent, cell-mediated cytotoxicity (ADCC) mechanisms may be involved in cellular immunity by recognition of viral agents on the membranes of infected cells. For certain groups of viruses, infection or immunization is known to stimulate lymphocytes which are cytotoxic for virus-infected target cells. The cytotoxic T lymphocyte (CTL) response is independent of antibody action. Cytotoxic T cell reactivity, though not proven to play a dominant role in prevention of infection, should be important in the recovery from diseases, particularly those involving obligate intracellular pathogens with non-infectious stages of replication. Recent studies in volunteers have, for instance, shown an association between high levels of influenza-specific CTL and rapid clearing of the virus after deliberate intranasal challenge with influenza virus. CTL activity cannot distinguish between different subtypes of influenza virus A, but might contribute to immunity toward different subtypes (108).

Natural killer (NK) cells are a class of cytotoxic leukocytes which non-specifically lyse various cell types, including virus-infected target cells. Increases in NK activity may at least in part be due to the stimulation of interferon production as a result of virus infection. For obligate intracellular pathogens (organisms that can live only inside cells), macrophage activation by lymphokines secreted by specific T cells would be the major host protective effector mechanism. Although at present there is no direct evidence that these cells are essential for immunity or recovery from viral infections, there are indications that some of them may specifically, or preferentially, kill certain virus-infected target cells.

The secretion of such mediators may be important for the efficacy and safety of vaccines and should be assessed when new vaccines are developed.

Section III – Consequences of Vaccines for Health and for Society

Introduction

As described in Section 2, vaccines are one of the most beneficial technologies available to the health care system. They are also technologies that are more involved with public policy decisions than other technologies. Traditionally, governments have made special efforts to develop vaccines. In the case of some vaccines, governments also make concerted attempts to encourage, or even require, their use. As biological products, vaccines are the subject of careful regulation to minimize risks and assure benefits.

In the Netherlands the mechanism by which this task is carried out, the Committee for the Regulation of Sera and Vaccines (Commissie ex artikel 14 Sera- en Vaccinsbesluit), was described in Volume I of the reports from this project and will not be analyzed further here.

Cost-Effectiveness of Vaccines

Cost-effectiveness analysis is a method of putting the costs of a program in relation to its benefits. Such a calculation is important in any program. It is particular critical in a public program with constrained resources. This fact probably explains why the cost-effectiveness of vaccines has been so frequently studied.

Cost-effectiveness analysis does not necessarily provide the definitive basis for a decision on vaccine use (120). The technique provides the decision-maker a structured framework for understanding the components of a decision and its subsequent effects. An analysis should force key assumptions to be made explicit and identify areas in which data are inadequate.

Ten vaccines have been examined for their cost-effectiveness. All are financial successes, in the sense that benefits, as valued, exceed costs for some target groups and in some situations. Still, almost all of the studies neglect some benefits, including quality of life and lost production of parents who miss work because of a disease in a child (162). In short, vaccines are even more cost-effective than indicated by the literature. This report will focus on measles (8 studies); pneumonia (5 studies); mumps (4 studies); rubella (6 studies); influenza (4 studies); polio (2 studies); pertussis (2 studies); and hepatitis B (1 study).

For measles, despite some problems in the studies, the eight studies all indicate that social benefits far outweigh social costs (2;5;46;91;98;99;164;167). These studies use a number of different time periods and examine Austria, Finland, and the United States. Witte and Axnick (167) may be taken as an example. They found that net savings from measles immunization in the United States were US$1.3 billion during the period 1963-1972. Benefits were approximately five times as large as the costs.

The studies of polio vaccine show it to be highly cost-effective (53;162). The Fudenberg results have been presented earlier.

Pertussis vaccine has been the subject of two studies (70;90). The Hinman and Koplan study (70) is an update of the earlier Koplan et al (90) analysis. They used a hypothetical cohort of children followed from birth to the age of 6 years old. The societal cost was found to be US$53.5 million without a program and US$9.5 million with the program. The benefit-cost ratio (reduction in disease costs divided by program costs) was 11 to 1. It should be noted that this analysis included the best available data on the complications of pertussis vaccine (see discussion of future vaccine possibilities in the next section).

The studies of mumps all show financial savings (98;99;89;164). Koplan and Preblud (89) carried out the most comprehensive analysis. In their results, each cohort of 1 million children vaccinated produces a net benefit of US$5 million. The ratio of benefits to costs was 7.4.

Rubella has been the subject of six studies (47;48;91;98;99;144). This program is also beneficial. The Schoenbaum et al (144) study has a comprehensive analysis, especially of benefits. The ratio of benefits to costs is found to be 8 to 1 if all 2 year old females are vaccinated, 9 to 1 if all 6 year old females are vaccinated, and 27 to 1 if all 12 year old females are vaccinated.

Influenza vaccine has been the subject of four studies (83;118;145; 152). All analyses find it to be cost-effective, but benefits exceed costs only for high risk persons. The Office of Technology Assessment did a very comprehensive analysis of this vaccine and found it to be cost-effective (118). The average cost of increasing healthy life expectancy ranged from about US$2,000 in the worst case to money saving in persons over the age of 44 in the best set of assumptions.

Pneumococcal vaccine has been the subject of five studies (31;34;122; 127;165). These studies find the vaccine cost-saving only when used in high-risk groups. The Willems et al study (165), published in longer form by the US Government Printing Office (121), is interesting because it led the U.S. Congress to cover the vaccine under the Medicare program. The cost of a quality adjusted life year was found to be US$1,000 for those over the age of 65.

Finally, Mulley et al (107) carried out an analysis of the costs and benefits of the hepatitis B vaccine marketed beginning in 1982. With little experience to go on, the investigators were forced to be very speculative, and analyzed alternative vaccination strategies for different population groups. The problem with this vaccine, from the standpoint of cost-effectiveness analysis, is that it is very expensive. It is therefore more difficult for the vaccine to be cost-effective. The analysis found that the most effective strategy for vaccinating homosexual men, a high risk group, was to screen for hepatitis antibodies first, and then give the vaccine only to those with no antibodies. This alternative cost about US$66 per person, compared with about US$100 per person for vaccinating all. For a medium risk population, surgical residents of hospitals, vaccinating everyone was the lowest cost option, costing about US$104 per person. However, for those countries with a high prevalence of hepatitis B and liver cancer, the calculations may be quite different. Wider use of this vaccine seems to depend on lowering its cost (162).

A benefit-cost analysis is being done of a proposed future vaccine, to Hemophilus influenzae (87). Preliminary analysis suggests that net benefit would occur if the vaccine had a 90 percent efficacy for one and one-half year's duration, vaccine acceptance rate of 80 percent, was useful only in children 18 months of age and older, cost US$3 per dose, and was given to all children accepting it 18 months and over. With a cohort of 3.6 million children, US$8,8 million in vaccination program costs would avert US$11 million in disease costs (30).

A 1985 report from the U.S. Institute of Medicine (74) gives detailed estimates for disease burdens and costs for a variety of diseases that may in the future be preventable by immunization.

In summary, vaccines are some of the most cost-effective interventions available in health care. There are few health care technologies that can reduce health care costs, but vaccines, applied to the optimal population group, are one example.

Factors in Utilization of Vaccines

The cost-effectiveness of a vaccine is not the only factor in determining whether it will be used. Even if social policy is to encourage a certain vaccine, physicians and patients must be willing to accept it.

Factors affecting utilization of a vaccine include the following (74):
1. vaccine availability;
2. The effects of statutory interventions, such as school immunization requirements (see later);
3. characteristics of the target population, including its access to health care providers;
4. characteristics of the vaccine that may affect the provider, including route of administration, storage conditions, cost of delivery, and special procedures required;
5. characteristics of the vaccine that may affect patient acceptance (number of doses, route of administration, adverse reactions, and cost; and
6. target population attitudes toward the vaccine.

Factors that physicians may consider in assessing a patient's need for a particular vaccine include (121, p. 181):
1. the likelihood of the patient's being exposed to the particular organism;
2. the patient's vulnerability to the disease once exposed to the organism; and
3. the extent to which contracting the disease will cause mortality or morbidity or disrupt the patient's life.

A particular problem is the data base that physicians use to make these judgments. For old vaccines and well-controlled diseases, data are generally available and physicians are familiar with them through their training. For new vaccines, however, physicians rely on traditional sources of information, including peers and professional literature. Vaccines are not generally actively promoted by industry. Government may not take an active role in education. Perhaps these factors explain why physician acceptance of a new vaccine may be quite low (126).

Recently, awareness of complications of vaccines has been growing, and some countries, such as the United States, have faced the problem of compensation for vaccine-related injury. Publicity surrounding this problem may have discouraged physicians from prescribing new vaccines (117;121, p. 181).

If the physician recommends a vaccine, the lay person must still accept it. Acceptance of a vaccine depends on such factors as (121, p. 175):

1. perception of the danger of the particular disease;
2. beliefs regarding the efficacy and safety of the vaccine; and
3. the convenience of being vaccinated.

A factor that seems more important in recent years for lay people as well as providers is the perceived risk of vaccines. The 1976 experience in the United States with the emergency vaccination program for swine influenza eroded public confidence in new vaccines (88). The fact that hepatitis B vaccine was made from serum has led to fears that it might be a carrier of AIDS. The release of the recombinant DNA hepatitis B vaccine (see below) ends this potential threat. However, can the average member of the public make a realistic assessment of risks?

Negative publicity around a vaccine may have serious consequences. An example is the rapid fall in coverage with pertussis vaccine, especially in the United Kingdom and the Federal Republic of Germany after dramatic publicity concerning the adverse reactions of this vaccine. In Sweden and Japan, pertussis vaccination had been officially stopped. In these countries, pertussis disease (whooping cough) reoccurred, producing far more damage and even death than the side effects of the vaccine. In the Netherlands, the authorities have warned against the reoccurence of the disease, and as a consequence coverage with pertussis vaccine did not drop below 90 percent.

The Institute of Medicine (74) has judged provider and consumer acceptance of a wide variety of possible future vaccines, using the categories risk, severity, benefits, and barriers.

The new biotechnology could improve acceptance of vaccines in a number of ways. One would be to produce safer vaccines, with minimal adverse reactions. Another would be to produce polytopic vaccines containing immunologically important parts of several organisms, cutting down the number of vaccine administrations. As an example, a new acellular pertussis vaccine is in preparation in several laboratories, including the RIVM. Finally, development of new methods of administration of vaccines, such as nasal sprays and oral vaccines, could play a role.

The effect of the cost of vaccination on vaccine acceptance has not been assessed. One must assume that the cost of hepatitis B vaccine - in the Netherlands about Dfl 200 per course of 3 injections - affects utilization. The desirability of vaccines from the standpoint of public health has often led to provision of vaccines free of charge.

Social Policy Toward Vaccines

Rates of immunization in the population have varied rather dramatically over time, and are related to a number of factors. Some of these factors have been discussed above. Since vaccines are preventive measure whose benefits occur sometime in the future and are not dramatic, they may not be sought as actively as other health care technologies.

The importance of social policy in vaccine use may be illustrated by the case of measles vaccine in the United States. When the Federal government has provided money for measles vaccine, the number of immunizations has risen, and the number of cases of measles has fallen. When the Federal government has not provided money, the number of immunizations has fallen and the number of cases of measles has risen (121, p. 183).

Because of this fact, and because high rates of immunization are necessary to prevent epidemics, governments have provided vaccines as part of their public health programs. As already noted, vaccines have been the classic case for the application of cost-effectiveness analysis in public health care expenditures. Analyses have shown again and again that vaccines are very good investments, often actually saving the society resources.

Governments often require certain immunizations among their population, especially for children entering school. A typical requirement is that a child would be required to be immunized against tetanus, diphtheria, pertussis, measles, rubella, and mumps. The vaccines are generally provided free or at low cost through public health programs.

For vaccines against diseases prevalent in the adult population, the situation is not so positive. The two main vaccines in question are influenza vaccine and pneumococcal vaccine (mainly to prevent bacterial pneumonia). These vaccines are provided sporadically through public health programs, and few countries have achieved high rates of immunization against these problems (88). In the United States, where pneumococcal vaccine is provided to all elderly people through the Medicare program, immunization rates nonetheless continue at a low level.

In the future, new vaccines will encounter similar problems of acceptance by professionals and the public alike. New vaccines against childhood diseases are much more likely to be accepted than others, since the child is under active physician surveillance and the mother makes most health care decisions. Otherwise, vaccines will not be given to the entire population of a certain age, but only to those at risk. The problem may be illustrated by the case of a vaccine against gonorrhea. The population at risk must not only be identified, but must in some way be convinced to seek and accept the vaccine.

In the future, governments may need to consider much more active attempts to 'educate' the public concerning vaccines. In short, if the government of a country is convinced, by cost-effectiveness analyses or other studies, that a vaccine should be widely used, will it seek to influence behavior of the public? If so, how will such attempts be developed and structured?

Section IV – The Netherlands Situation

Introduction

This section provides a brief description of the public and private participants in present-day vaccine development, production, supply, and utilization in the Netherlands.

For the development of new generations of vaccines, a number of scientific disciplines have to work together. These disciplines include immunology, molecular biology, structural- and bio-chemistry, and bioprocess technology. In the Netherlands, these disciplines are available in universities, state institutes, institutes of applied research, and industry.

Vaccine Development, Production and Use

The most important Dutch institute involved in the development and production of vaccines is the National Institute of Public Health and Environmental Hygiene (RIVM). In the Netherlands, vaccines for use in The National Vaccination Programs are all made in this institution (56) (see Table 3). Vaccines are produced for three target populations:

1. The National Vaccination Program for children
2. The Military Vaccination Program
3. Travellers Vaccination Program

The National Vaccination Program consists of a fourfold vaccination of siblings with a combined Diphtheria, Tetanus, Pertussis, and Polio (DTP-Polio) vaccine, and further booster vaccinations of children at four and nine years of age. Since 1987 a combined measles, mumps, and rubella (MMR) vaccine is given at 14 months of age, with a repeat vaccination at nine years of age. For the Military Vaccination Program and for travellers, both typhoid vaccine and cholera vaccine are prepared. For a small target population of people with a high risk of tuberculosis, the BCG vaccine is prepared. For the treatment of people infected by an animal suspected of rabies, an inactivated rabies vaccine is produced. This inactivated rabies vaccine is safe enough so that, in contrast to the previous vaccines, it may also be used for the prevention of rabies in high risk situations.

Table 3 Vaccines produced by the RIVM

BCG	(Bacillus Calmette Guerin)
BMR (in development)	mumps, measles, and rubella
Cholera	
DPT-polio	diphtheria, pertussis, tetanus, and poliomyelitis
DTP	diphtheria, tetanus, and poliomyelitis
Diphtheria toxoid	
Tetanus toxoid	
Measles	(will be BMR)
Poliomyelitis	
Rabies	
Rubella	
Staphylococcus toxoid	
Typhoid	
Stock vaccines and auto vaccines	

Other institutes are also involved in the development and production of vaccines, though not at this large a scale. A number of universities are involved in fundamental research on immunological processes. For instance, research on third and fourth generation synthetic vaccines is done at the universities of Leiden, Nijmegen and Groningen. Often these studies are conducted in close collaboration with industry. The university of Leiden and Organon, for instance, are working together in the development of a Hemophilus vaccine. TNO is working on the development of a recombinant polio-vaccine.

RIVM limits itself to the production of vaccines that are in the National Vaccination Program. Other producers include The Central Laboratory of the Blood Transfusion Services (CLB), which is producing a plasma-derived hepatitis B vaccine. Commercial producers include: Duphar, Behring, and Pasteur for Influenza vaccine; Merck Sharp and Dome (MSD) for Pneumococcus vaccine; and Wellcome for yellow fever vaccine.

The classical preparation of vaccines was mainly done by small-scale non-automated laboratory processes, not allowing for standardization and automation of the production process. It gave rise to many risks of contamination. The introduction of the fermentation cultures in the 1960's gave rise to the standardization of the process and allowed for scaling up of the production. The fermentation technology was primarily applied to the cultivation of bacterial cells like Diphtheria, Tetanus, Pertussis, Cholera, Typhoid, and BCG. It resulted in the construction of an apparatus called the 'Bilthoven unit'. Growth takes place in a so called 'homogenous culture', in which the particles are homogenously distributed in a stirred suspension.

A further breakthrough was the application of the 'Bilthoven unit' in the production of viral vaccines. A problem in virus production is the fact that the cells used to grow the virus on do not multiply in suspension but only on a surface. The use of 'microcarriers' that can be kept in suspension solved this problem. This is a very good and widely used method in the production of inactivated vaccines. In the RIVM this method is now being applied to the production of polio and rabies vaccine. Application of the technique leads to a reduced need of primary cells and reduces production costs.

The new biotechnology is fully incorporated in RIVM's vaccine development. The vaccinia approach is being exploited for HIV vaccine development, synthetic protein subunits are being developed for HIV, measles, and rabies, and the potential of anti-idiotype vaccines is being studied in polioviruses, rabies virus, canine parvovirus, feline leukemia virus, and HIV (the cause of AIDS). Within RIVM, a great amount of work has been aimed at improving the antigenicity of viral vaccines, primarily aiming at subunit vaccine development for rabies virus, measles virus, feline leukemia virus (model 4), and HIV.

The same techniques used in growing cell cultures are applicable to many other fields of biotechnology. The large-scale production of monoclonal antibodies and enzymes is now possible by applying fermentation technology. Within RIVM, much attention has been paid to this upscaling procedure of in-vitro monoclonal antibody production.

Within the RIVM, monoclonal antibodies are being used for several research applications, especially in the field of infectious (viral, bacterial, and parasitic) diseases and immunology. Many epidemiological studies have been conducted with monoclonal antibodies. They also are being used to study the relationships between structure and function in various viruses. The applicability of monoclonal antibodies for vaccine production, as in immune affinity purification, developments in anti-idiotype vaccines, and vaccine control, as in potency and safety tests, is the subject of intense study. As a result monoclonal antibodies already have been introduced in many routine procedures. Finally, monoclonals against specific T-cell markers are made for functional studies.

At RIVM the diagnostic potential of monoclonal antibodies has been exploited in a great number of fields. Diagnostic tests incorporating monoclonal antibodies have been made for the diagnosis of infections with: polioviruses; rabies virus; herpes viruses (HSV1/HSV2); influenza viruses; measles virus; adenoviruses (types 40/41); AIDS virus; mouse hepatitis virus; avian leukaemia virus; bovine leukemia virus; feline leukemia virus; canine parvovirus; canine distemper virus; infectious bronchitis virus; Treponema pallidum (the cause of syphilis); Neisseria meningitidis; Escherichia coli (K99, F41, P987); Salmonella species; and Mycoplasma species. Some of these have been or are being incorporated in diagnostic kits. Another kit incorporates a number of monoclonal antibodies that are generated against human T-cell markers.

Anti T-cell monoclonal antibodies are also being investigated at RIVM for therapeutic use in immunosuppression. Anti-rabies virus and anti-measles virus monoclonal antibodies are being tested for potential use in post-exposure treatment. A third program on therapautic applications concerns the development of anti-tumor markers for cancer treatment.

The RIVM is actively involved in transferring its production technology to developing countries for the development of large scale local production processes of vaccines. An already existing example is the large scale production process of rabies vaccine developed with aid of WHO and other international organizations. Dutch industry is supplying the necessary equipment for the production plants in the projects.

Priorities for Future Vaccine Development

The United States Institute of Medicine examined the potentials for vaccine development in 1985 (74). Using a complex formula involving predictions of target population, efficacy, vaccine cost, anticipated utilization rate, and so forth, the IOM ranked the possible vaccines in order of importance. If only expected health benefit is considered, these are the top five for the U.S. population:

- Hepatitis B
- Respiratory syncytial virus (a cause of upper respiratory infections)
- Hemophilus influenzae B (a cause of infections, including ear infections, in children)
- Influenza
- Herpesvirus varicellae (high risk individuals only)

Acquired Immunodeficiency Syndrome (AIDS) was excluded from consideration by the Institute of Medicine group because of the large amount of activity already underway concerning this epidemic disease. The Institute of Medicine has carried out separate reports dealing specifically with AIDS (73).

In the Netherlands, options for the application of new vaccines have been traditionally discussed in the appropriate committees of the Health Council (Gezondheidsraad). This sometimes led to the introduction of a new vaccine in the National Immunization Program. The publication of **New Vaccine Development** by the Institute of Medicine (74) gave an impetus for the development of a priority ranking system of vaccines specific for the situation in the Netherlands. RIVM has considered developing such a system in close collaboration with the Netherlands Institute for Preventive Medicine (NIPG).

Consequences for Health: Vaccine Cases

To illustrate the importance of developments in biotechnology for vaccine development, and for potential health benefits for the population of the Netherlands, seven cases of diseases affecting the Dutch population are presented, along with information on the prospects for new or improved vaccines in each case. Three groups of diseases are presented: those for which vaccines are already available; those for which vaccines are being tested; and those for which vaccines yet have to be developed.

Bordetella pertussis. This organism, a bacterium, causes the disease known as pertussis or whooping cough, a disease seriously affecting mainly infants and young children. The main characteristic of the disease is severe, continued coughing that may persist for weeks. Complications of the disease include encephalopathy (brain infection/damage) and convulsions, pulmonary atelectasis (collapse of part of the lung), and secondary infections such as pneumonia and otitis media (middle ear infection) (105). The major cause of death from whooping cough arises from secondary infections such as pneumonia (79). Whooping cough is still responsible for a significant number of deaths in infants in areas where pertussis immunization is not practiced (79).

Treatment with antibiotics is not very successful with pertussis. When the treatment is started very early it may have some effects on the symptoms. The major advantage, however, is the inhibition of the infectious process.

A vaccine for pertussis was introduced about 1914, and it has been part of the standard package of childhood immunizations in the Netherlands since 1953, along with diphtheria and tetanus vaccines (DPT vaccine). In 1962 DTP-vaccine was replaced by DTP-Polio vaccine. From then on, over 90% of all newborns received a complete immunization (62;63). The vaccine is composed of inactivated cells of the organism. It is given four times, beginning at the age of 3 months, and induces good immunity against the disease. It is about 90 percent effective in preventing the disease (25). Widespread application of the vaccine led to a rapid decline in the incidence of the disease. In the 1940s, for example, there were about 200,000 cases reported annually in the United States; in the late 1970s, fewer than 2,000 a year were reported (79). In the period 1940-1946 a mean number of 463 children died annually from pertussis in the Netherlands. From 1964 on, no children died from pertussis. The number of reported cases dropped to less than 30 annually (63), although after 1980 a gradual increase is found. At the same time, the disease might not disappear completely as the bacterium may circulate among the healthy population without giving rise to typical symptoms of pertussis.

In recent years, the vaccine has become controversial because of complications of its administration. Low grade fever and tenderness at the site of injection are common. More or less severe reactions, including shock, convulsions, encephalopathy (signs of brain damage), and persistent high-pitched screaming, occur as rare complications (70). In the Netherlands the incidences of shock and convulsions are both about 1 in 2700 vaccinated children. Encephalopathy has an incidence of about 1 in 400.000 vaccinated children (63). Mental retardation can result in an estimated 6 cases per million (117). Fatal complications occur in an estimated 1 or 2 cases per 10 million injections (74, p. 173). Because of these complications, the use of the vaccine has declined in such countries as the United Kingdom, Japan, and Sweden. Disease rates have risen as a result of this decline. For example, the UK had an epidemic in 1977-1979 with more than 100.000 cases of pertussis and 28 deaths (79). The epidemic was repeated in 1981/82 and 1985/86. There seems little doubt that vaccination programs using the present vaccine are cost-effective (70). In other words, more illness and death occurs without the vaccine, when the disease rises in prevalence in the community.

Because of the rise in incidence of the disease in Japan, Japanese scientists developed an acellular vaccine, based mainly on two protein antigens that seem to induce a protective immune response. This vaccine has been used in Japan since 1980. Vaccination started at the age of two years and resulted in fewer reactions than the previous vaccination, starting at the age of three month. Its safety and efficacy has not yet been formally reported. It is being tested in a clinical trial in Sweden and is also being tested in the United States (74, p. 178). At the same time, work is going on in various countries, including the Netherlands, to develop similar alternative vaccines based on one or more of the virulence factors of B.pertussis. The Dutch development of an acellular pertussis vaccine is in an advanced stage; clinical trials using this vaccine are expected in 1987.

Research is in progress to study the virulence factors of B. pertussis at a molecular level. At the same time, studies on the pathogenesis of B. pertussis infection infection have led to the detection of the subcellular components which are responsible for the acquisition of protective immunity against infection.

The importance of a non-reactogenic pertussis vaccine is that the public of several countries has tended to reject the vaccine, resulting in a rising incidence of complications and deaths caused by the disease. A vaccine with severe reactions can undermine public confidence in the entire public health vaccination program.

Influenza. Influenza is a viral disease that is a widespread problem in industrialized countries. Influenza is characterized by nasal congestion, sore throat, hoarseness, and cough, as well as fever, muscle aches and pains, and malaise (feeling of tiredness) (55;74, p. 342). Severe cough is fairly frequent. Although influenza is generally considered to be a mild disease, it is also associated with pneumonia and death in some cases, particularly in the elderly and in those with chronic lung problems, particularly children with cystic fibrosis. Influenza is the greatest cause of excess mortality (mortality in excess of the baseline) in western societies (26).

Influenza is passed from person to person. It usually occurs in the winter and can either occur sporadically or in epidemic form. Most interest focuses on one strain, Influenza A, which tends to be associated with epidemics (82). Periodically, worldwide epidemics (pandemics) tend to occur, in which the virus spreads very rapidly through the world and almost all cases of respiratory tract illness are attributable to influenza virus.

A natural case of influenza induces effective immunity against that strain. The problem is that the immunity is to two glycoproteins (antigens) in the surface of the virus. These surface antigens change frequently, and when they change greatly from the previous strain, immunity is no longer effective. Such 'antigenic shifts' explain in part the development of periodic epidemics (37). The immune response to the virus and the nature of immunity is not completely understood (74, 344).

A vaccine was produced in 1945 against the influenza virus, using virus grown in embryonated eggs and then chemically inactivated. Viruses can now be grown in several types of cell culture (74, 343). The vaccine gives good protection against the particular strain of the virus. Nonetheless, the antigenic shifts make it necessary to reformulate the vaccine and administer it annually for good control of the disease in the population. The need for annual revaccinations, misconceptions about the capabilities of the vaccines, and unanswered questions about efficacy in high-risk populations have led both the public and professionals to the frequent attitude that influenza vaccine is not worth the effort (74, p. 342).

Present work on improving available vaccines focuses on two possibilities. One is to improve the currently available inactivated vaccines. The other is to develop a live attenuated virus vaccine that will grow only in the upper respiratory tract (but not in the lung) and that would be given by nasal drops (29;156). Such a virus might be associated with longer immunity (82). It is also possible to make vaccines containing antigens of disrupted virus. Other possibilities including the non-specific responses in the respiratory tract occurring just after infection and the role of specific cytotoxic T-cells, which appear to be crucial for recovery, are also being investigated. The designed vaccine should both limit the occurrence of the infection and also provide priming at the cellular level to assist in recovery from infection. Interesting for influenza vaccine development, as well as for some other viruses and a number of parasites, is the potential possibility of overcoming the antigenic variation by using antigens located on constant regions. However, no evidence yet supports the feasibility of this approach.

General population immunization against influenza is not indicated, because of the usually mild nature of the disease (82). Reconsideration of this principle depends on having a more effective and safe vaccine. The goal at the moment is to develop a vaccine that can prevent the disease in elderly and high-risk people. However, given negative attitudes toward the vaccine, acceptance in any case may be a long-term problem (74. p 358). An added factor complicating possible acceptance is the nasal route of administration of a possible new attenuated vaccine, a route not generally familiar to the population.

Hepatitis B. Hepatitis B virus causes acute hepatitis (inflammation of the liver). In many cases, the infection causes no symptoms, but it can also be characterized by nausea, vomiting, abdominal pain, generalized aching, a rash, and jaundice (114). Severe cases may require hospitalization and death can follow the severe form of the disease. Approximately 10 percent of adults infected develop a chronic carrier state for the virus, which can be associated with symptoms, but also can leave the person seemingly healthy (114). It is estimated that there are 200 million carriers of human hepatitis B virus in the world (3;174). Chronic infection can be followed, years later, by cirrhosis of the liver or liver carcinoma (13).

It is estimated that about 200,000 cases a year occur in the United States (74, p. 263) yielding about 20,000 new carriers; this corresponds to almost 14,000 cases a year and 1,400 new carriers in the Netherlands. Of these carriers, about one in five die of liver cirrhosis, and one in twenty die of liver carcinoma (3;52).

The hepatitus B virus is most often transmitted parenterally (e.g. by needles), through intimate sexual contact, or perinatally from infected mothers to their newborn infants. Groups at high risk from parenteral exposure include health care personnel who have contact with blood; drug addicts; and people receiving multiple blood transfusions. High risk individuals include homosexuals with multiple sex partners and sex partners of those with acute or chronic infection. Only about half of the cases occur in high risk groups, however (74, p. 266).

People develop immunity to the hepatitis B virus (97). The development of a conventional vaccine has been hampered by the failure to grow hepatitis B virus in tissue culture. Because of this fact other preparations which might produce active immunity were sought. Workers in different countries, including the United States, France, and the Netherlands, developed effective plasma-derived hepatitis B vaccines (23;36;58;67;137). It has been available since 1982 and is licensed and recommended in several countries for routine use in high-risk populations (155). However, acceptance of the vaccine has been low, partly because of its high cost and perhaps partly because of concerns about its source (plasma from donors who may be at risk of other infections).

Alternate approaches to vaccine development that partially solve this problem include use of a hepatitis B surface antigen (HBsAg)-producing hepatocellular carcinoma (HCC) cell line, recombinant DNA technology, and in vitro creation of synthetic peptides (7;96). The major barrier for HCC cell line vaccine is the general concern about using a cancer cell line for vaccine production. In recombinant technology the HBsAg genome is inserted into a plasmid which in turn is inserted into a bacterium, yeast, cultured mammalian cells, or another virus (104;150; 160). With bacterial and yeast recombinant vaccines, HBsAg is incorporated into the cell membrane or cell wall and cellular components must be removed to obtain purified HBsAg. In 1986, a new (yeast) recombinant Hepatitus B vaccine was registered in the United States and West Germany. Its success is not yet known.

It should be remembered that yeast recombinant antigen is the same antigen as that derived from human plasma and therefor offers no clinical advantage for efficacy (67). Potential advantages include the limitless supply, fewer side-effects, and perhaps most important, the availability of a model for developing future vaccines against other viruses for which there is no other means for antigen preparation. In virus recombinant vaccines, the gene for hepatitis B surface antigen is inserted into the vaccinia virus gene. The virus replicates in animals, and antibody to hepatitis B surface antigen is generated in response to the hepatitis B surface antigen that is produced. However, the use of vaccinia as a vector has certain drawbacks, (see section 2; viral vectors).

Plans are being made by the World Health Organization to map a strategy for eventual eradication of hepatitis B from the world population by vaccination (100). The strategy is seen mainly as a cancer prevention program (13;175). The high cost of the vaccine, however, is a barrier to the success of this strategy.

Haemophilus influenzae type b. Haemophilus influenzae type b (Hib) is a bacterium that causes disease of the upper respiratory tract and the bronchopulmonary tree (bronchi and lungs). It is a major cause of meningitis and other serious complications, which occur mainly in young children between the ages of 6 months and one year (158). (Other types of the bacterium cause little serious illness.) Neurological problems, including hearing and vision loss, problems in the motor (movement) system, seizure disorders, severe mental retardation, and paralysis may follow a case of meningitis (111). The incidence of meningitis from this cause was estimated to be 9,000 cases in the United States (74, p. 237), corresponding to about 600 cases a year in the Netherlands. However, the actual Dutch figures appear to be lower. The incidence of other invasive infections, including pneumonia, was estimated to be about 5,000 cases in the United States.

Hib does not cause epidemics in the population. One issue of concern is that in USA day care centers an increased incidence of Hib diseases has been demonstrated (74, p. 240).

The disease can be effectively treated with antibiotics if the treatment is begun early. However, even with treatment, chronic neurological symptoms often occur after recovery (74,p. 240). Many strains of the organism have become resistant to antibiotics such as ampicillin (158).

The organism causes an effective immune response. Antibodies are induced to both proteins of the surface of the organisms and to its capsular polysaccharide. The fact that disease is seldom seen to occur twice in the same child and in children over the age of 5 years is evidence of long-lasting immunity (74, p. 236). A vaccine has been developed using the capsular polysaccharide, and it has been shown to be protective in children over 24 months of age in a clinical trial in Finland (130;131). However, unfortunately, it was not protective against the disease in children below the age of 18 months (158). A vaccine is needed that is protective for younger children (74, p. 236). Current developments focus on a polysaccharide-protein conjugate vaccine. The polysaccharide is combined with a protein carrier, which improves the antigenic response. The first results of use in siblings are very promising.

Haemophilus influenzae disease is well-suited for control by vaccination because the antibody seems to provide protection and it seems likely that such protection can be induced between the ages of 3 and 6 months, prior to the peak incidence of the disease. It is estimated that 90 percent of the illness in the first year of life is potentially preventable by one or more injection of the vaccine, beginning at the age of 2-3 months (74, p. 238).

The acceptance of the vaccine would probably be good because physicians have a relatively accurate idea of the severity of the disease. The vaccine could and may be incorporated in the National Immunization Programme of the Netherlands.

Herpes simplex viruses 1 and 2 (HSV). These viruses cause a wide variety of diseases, ranging from inapparent infections and 'fever blisters' to fatal encephalitis (brain infection) (40). Lesions of the skin and mucous membranes are characteristic of infection.

The two types of the virus cause problems at different sites. HSV-2 traditionally has been regarded as a virus transmitted primarily by sexual contact or by the mother to the baby during birth . Approximately 1 in 7,500 live births show neonatal HSV-1 (35). It usually occurs at body sites above the waist, mostly the mouth, and is most common in childhood. Infection can be without symptoms, but can also be accompanied by severe disease.

Infection is complicated by the fact that the virus is retained (latent) in nervous tissue for life and may cause recurrences of the disease periodically (40). The disease is most often severe and generalized when it occurs in people with problems of their immune system (those being treated with drugs for cancer, for example) and in newborns. Infections of the eye can lead to blindness and infection of the brain (encephalitis) can be fatal. Type 2 has been linked to cervical cancer in women (74, p. 280).

The form of the disease that has been most publicized is genital herpes. The U.S. Institute of Medicine estimated a cumulative incidence of genital herpes in the United States of 15 percent by age

35 (74, p. 283). IOM also estimated that each case will have an average of two recurrences per year.

Treatment of herpes is not very successful. Chemotherapeutic agents do control primary infection, but they do not prevent the establishment of the latent virus (74, p. 292).

Herpes viruses provoke an immune response, encouraging the idea that a vaccine is possible. Infection with the virus is followed by development of an antibody that persists for life (40). However, these antibodies do not prevent recurrence of latent infection. Thus, it will probably be necessary to develop immunity prior to exposure to the virus to achieve protection (74, p. 281)

The goal is to develop a vaccine for administration in infancy or early childhood to prevent or reduce the replication of virus during primary infection (74, p. 291). The immunity level would have to be high to prevent the virus from establishing latency. This would mean repeated injections of a subunit vaccine (74, p. 292). This raises particular problems in young adults.

Work has proceeded on herpes vaccines for years without much success. Recent work has focused on the use of glycoprotein surface antigens administered with an adjuvant (68;161). Such vaccines induce antibody formation in humans, and they are now being tested in clinical trials. In addition, it is possible to use recombinant DNA technology to produce a live virus vaccine, which should produce longer-lasting immunity (74, p. 300). Another approach to vaccine development has utilized rDNA technology to incorporate the viral gene coding for protective glycoproteins into vaccinia virus and then to immunize with the modified hybrid vaccinia virus (109). If a vaccine were developed and proven, it would probably have a fair chance of finding widespread acceptance (74, p. 301). In the Netherlands research activities on HSV are limited to basic research at the University of Rotterdam.

Acquired Immunodeficiency Syndrome (AIDS). AIDS was discovered in 1981 and since then, reported cases have increased exponentially in a number of countries, including the Netherlands (73). Recent estimates suggest that up to one million Americans may have been exposed to the AIDS virus. Reported cases are only the tip of the iceberg, representing the full spectrum of infection with the human immunodeficiency virus (HIV). Patients with AIDS have a profound and selective depletion of a subpopulation of immune competent cells called helper T lymphocytes, which are responsible for the orchestration of the entire immune response in man. The entire spectrum of the disease includes asymptomatic infection; mild illness with such symptoms as fever, tiredness, loss of appetite and weight, diarrhea, and enlarged lymph nodes; and severe cellular immunodeficiency that leads the infected person to be prone to infection with a wide variety of agents that ordinarily do not cause human disease and threaten his or her life. The most common and one of the most serious of these is infection with Pneumocystis carinii (49). The infected person is also prone to malignancy, particularly Kaposi's sarcoma and lymphoma of the brain.

The long-term prognosis of those with the milder forms of the disease is not known. Persistent human infection is quite common. Observations suggest that 5 to 20 percent of these people will develop AIDS within 5 years of infection (41)

The causative virus was isolated in 1983 and 1984 (8). It has been recovered from blood, semen, and saliva. The virus is transmitted sexually or through exposure to blood or its components, including certain blood products. The virus has also been transmitted from infected mothers to their infants before, at, or shortly after birth (41). There is no evidence of household transmission and health care workers have not been found to be at high risk. Those most at risk include homosexual men, hemophiliacs, intravenous drug abusers, and transfusion recipients (41;139). In the Netherlands, however, the risk of blood transfusion recipients has dropped since screening-tests and virus inactivation of plasma products were introduced.

There is no treatment of the disease itself. The resulting (secondary) infections however, can be treated with drugs. Malignancy can be treated with chemotherapy or radiation. The case-fatality rate of the disease is high, with about 85 percent dead within three years of diagnosis (41).

Prevention at the moment depends on education of high-risk groups. Recommendations for prevention of AIDS are deceptively easy: avoid sex with those known or suspected of being infected and use condoms when having different partners; stop using intravenous drugs or avoid sharing drug administration equipment; eliminate infected blood from use in transfusions. Sexual habits have already changed as a result of AIDS. For instance, the use of condoms as preventive measure has increased in the last few years. Still, changing behavior is difficult in practice.

A vaccine could be developed. The genome of the causal retrovirus has been extensively characterized, and a number of groups have reported the expression of viral proteins in bacteria as well as vaccinia virus (81;136). A major obstacle in the development a vaccine to HIV, however, is the variability of the virus, which may present serious obstacles to the generation of broadly effective immunity. Vaccine development is also constrained by the presently limited basic understanding of the immune response to HIV infection (73). A potential lead that has not been explored in detail is the cellular response to virally infected cells. Since the cellular arm of the immune response is thought to be most relevant to the elimination of virally infected cells, its recruitment may be the most effective target for vaccination strategies (163). The most likely approach to an HIV vaccine is through the discovery of broadly protective immunizing antigens and epitopes and their expression by recombinant DNA technology. As the candidate immunogens, including the external glycoproteins, are heavily glycosylated, mammalian cells are probably required for production (73). Recently, the production of a large segment of the HIV envelope glycoprotein has been achieved in mammalian tissue cells (16). RIVM is involved in the isolation of HIV antigens, at this stage for diagnostic purposes but possibly later also for vaccine development. An additional effort of RIVM is the development of epidemiological models of AIDS, to be used when testing a vaccine.

Passive immunization by the administration of specific immunoglobulins, prepared from plasma of immunized donors, should be mentioned as well. These immunoglobulins have already been used for many years for the prevention of infectious diseases like hepatitis B, tetanus, rubella, etc. At present, a joint effort of institutes in Paris, New York, and the Netherlands (CLB) is attempting to develop an immunoglobulin concentrate containing neutralizing antibodies to HIV which could be of use for the prevention of its transmission.

Identification of high-risk groups, and convincing them to accept the vaccine, probably will raise problems for a vaccination program.

Cytomegalovirus. Cytomegalovirus is a virus that is a frequent cause of inapparent infections that can cause disease at any age. Its importance, however, is due to infections of the fetus in utero, with associated irreversible damage to the central nervous system (64). An estimated 1 percent of fetuses are infected, making cytomegalovirus infection the most common known fetal infection (64;74, p. 200). Only 5 to 10 percent of these infections cause symptoms, but 1 or 2 percent of these are fatal. Almost 90 percent of the infections leave the survivors with (congenital) health problems. Cytomegalic inclusion disease (CID) is characterized by enlarged liver and spleen, jaundice, small hemorrhages in the skin (petechiae), pneumonia, and infection of the eye (chorioretinitis). Central nervous system symptoms and other neurological problems may be present at birth.

In addition, about 15 percent of congenitally infected infants who are asymptomatic at birth later develop chronic neurological problems, including hearing loss, minimal brain damage, and learning and behavioral disorders (74, p. 200-201).

Serious brain damage can result in complete paralysis and a complete vegetative state with no meaningful communication. Occasionally there are no specific symptoms, but the infant has increased irritability and failure to thrive (64).

The disease is not highly communicable, so some individuals remain susceptible into adult life. The virus is probably transferred by intimate contact with an infected individual or by infusion of blood from an asymptomatic blood donor (64).

There is no effective treatment for the disease.

There is also no effective vaccine against cytomegalovirus. There are barriers to developing an effective vaccine. Although the virus does provoke antibodies, these antibodies are not fully protective against infection. Even with antibodies, the person can continue to shed the virus for weeks or months, and latent infection often continues (74, p. 199). The disease can also be reactivated despite antibodies. In addition, the virus is a large and complicated one and its antigenic structure is not well understood.

It seems likely that a vaccine can be produced with recombinant DNA technology. The first necessity is to identify proteins of the virus that are associated with an immune response. If this can be done, the approach would probably be to identify and isolate the genes coding for these proteins. They could then be inserted into a host, such as a yeast, to produce the proteins. A vaccine based on these proteins would then need to be tested in animals and people (74, p. 225). The process will take some years.

The main recipient group for the vaccine would be nonpregnant adolescent females. How receptive this group would be to the vaccine is not known. In immuno-compromised patients, notably transplantation patients, a CMV-vaccine could be of use as well. The disease is not recognized in the population. On the other hand, a vaccine that promises to prevent mental retardation might have a high acceptance rate.

Setting Priorities in the Netherlands

In the project on future health care technology, an attempt was made, working with RIVM, to develop sound and complete information on the diseases specified above as an indication of priorities for vaccine development. Within the limits of the project in staff and time, it was not possible to develop a great deal of information. The main reason for this is the weak data collection systems concerning infectious diseases. Epidemiological analysis and monitoring systems are seriously deficient in the Netherlands, hampering efforts to determine appropriate strategies for vaccine development and use.

Section V – Conclusions

The field of biotechnology is developing rapidly. New research findings appear almost every day. The ultimate effect of the applications of this knowledge development is hard to foresee, but seems certain to be profound in a number of parts of society, such as agriculture. In the health care system, new preventive, diagnostic, and therapeutic tools - both in the short-run and the long-run - will surely lead to improved health. This report has highlighted the contribution of biotechnological techniques to research and development in the vaccine area.

One should not assume, however, that the main issue is the application of already existing tools. In fact, the main issue is the potentials for the future.

Conclusion 1. Research and development in the field of the new biotechnology deserves continued - and perhaps expanded - support. Periodic reports on the state of the art and on important fields for research support could be a valuable tool in developing policy toward research in this area.

The realization of new technologies resulting from biotechnology will depend primarily on long-term, stable research funding at adequate levels.

A second condition for success is that research is done in areas of most potential. The Health Council, as well as other groups, has already reported on possible advances in biotechnology. The Health Council's Commission on Health Biotechnology (Commissie Medische Biotechnologie) intends to continue this activity. No further action seems warranted in this area at this time.

Conclusion 2. The new biotechnology is also associated with real and potential social problems. Monitoring the overall situation could also be helpful in assuring that such problems are minimized.

The new biotechnology, like any other powerful new technology - is also associated with potential and real problems. Social consequences include effects on the health system, such as possible changes in the present structure of clinical laboratories and blood banks.

A particular development that might present problems is the development of diagnostic kits, and especially, their sale to the general public. At present, such direct sales are hardly regulated, since this has not been an important issue in the past. However, simplifications in tests that are developing from the field of biotechnology, especially those with monoclonal antibodies, makes a large number of kits possible. This may raise problems that need to be addressed in the future.

The remainder of the conclusions deal specifically with the field of vaccines:

Conclusion 3. In developing policy toward vaccines, continuing attention to strategies for vaccine development is needed. In particular, policies in any country need to be based on knowledge of efforts to develop vaccines in other countries.

Vaccines are among the most effective and cost-effective technologies available to the health care system. They protect against many diseases. They have prevented many millions of deaths and injuries.

Work in biotechnology and immunology promises great advances in the area of vaccines. Vaccines will be safer in the future, and new vaccines not previously possible will be developed. One problem is the use of research and development resources. What are the highest priorities in vaccine development?

For a country such as the Netherlands, it is impossible to develop all needed vaccines. In addition, the national market is too small to cover all research and development and production costs. Therefore, collaboration between institutions involved in vaccine development in different countries is an absolute requirement.

It could be useful to have more analysis of vaccine development strategies in the Netherlands. Efforts by RIVM and NIPG to develop a priority system for vaccines is a constructive step in this direction.

Conclusion 4. Information and data systems concerning infectious diseases potentially subject to control by vaccination need to be improved in the Netherlands.

This project has attempted to analyze the importance of vaccine development in several areas in the Netherlands. Information was not available on several significant diseases.

Rational planning for vaccine development and use requires knowledge of the extent and distribution of diseases in the population.

Conclusion 5. The effects of the new biotechnology on present policies toward vaccine use need to be examined.

Improved and more potent vaccines could result in simplification of immunization schedules, reducing demands on public health resources and, perhaps, improving social acceptance of vaccines. On the other hand, new vaccine developments raise certain problems that must be taken into account. (See next Conclusion)

Conclusion 6. Methods of orienting the public to the use of vaccines need more research. Research on factors promoting acceptance of vaccines could be beneficial in this respect. In particularly, the issue of selecting and motivating certain sub-groups of the public to accept a certain vaccine needs to be investigated. Publicity aimed at educating the public to the contribution of vaccines to health could be of benefit.

The acceptance of vaccines by the general public is of the utmost importance. Maintaining immunization rates against childhood disease above 90 percent, for example, totally prevents epidemics of childhood diseases that once ravaged the population. The highest priority should be given to maintaining such immunization rates.

Most vaccines in present use are given to all members of the population in a certain age group, usually children or the elderly. In the future, a number of new vaccines will have to be targeted to particular sub-groups in the population to be both effective and cost-effective. Behavioral science research specific to the question of acceptance of vaccines could be of value.

Conclusion 7. International efforts to eliminate disease through immunization need support. Elimination strategies should be formulated in larger geographic regions than individual countries whenever possible.

Infectious disease is not a national issue, but an international one, especially in Europe, with its small countries and its open borders. With better vaccines, improved control and even elimination of some diseases is feasible, but this will be most effective if done internationally.

Appendixes

APPENDIX A BIOLOGICAL RESPONSE MODIFIERS

Interferon is the first example of a widely available immunomodulator. Interferon proteins are natural molecules that are secreted following viral infection (142). Human cells produce at least a dozen different kinds of interferons, all of which are proteins (135). Until 1980 the sole source of human interferon was human cells. Vast quantities of white blood cells from donors were infected with viruses, stimulating them to produce, tiny amounts of, interferon. In 1980 the gene for one type of human interferon was successfully cloned and inserted into bacteria which promptly began manufacturing the substance. As a result these potent substances became the subject of the most widely publicized, well-funded applications of rDNA technology to date, although their effects remain somewhat questionable. Interferons have been considered for various applications, including treatment of viral infections and cancer (20;51). A role in viral infections seems possible because other, more specific, antiviral compounds are limited in their potential. For the treatment and prevention of the common cold, for example, which can be caused by 200 different (sub)types of viruses, specific chemotherapy will not be feasible. The development of general immune stimulants to treat the common cold, such as interferon or lymphokine-like substances, therefore, seems a more promising approach (102). Given as a prophylactic, in the form of a nasal spray, interferon appears to build resistance to common cold. Preliminary studies have revealed promising results in the treatment of rabies, hepatitis, shingles, various herpes infections and cytomegalovirus infections (135). However, the therapeutic effectiveness of interferons is yet unproven (20;22). Interferons in the treatment of cancer, especially certain leukemias and Kaposi's sarcoma, may be of benefit. A study reported in 1986 found interferon of benefit in multiple sclerosis (76).

In the long-run, interferon research may illuminate cellular function during immune responses. Without full knowledge of the function of the immune-apparatus in 'peace-time' and its operation in 'war-time, applications will be inherently limited. Through biotechnology more effective and cheaper methods of supplying interferon for research and, eventually, for a widespread use in medicine, come available.

Interleukin-2 (IL_2). T-cell growth factor (TCGF) or Interleukin-2 is one of the lymphokines produced by stimulating lymphocytes. Incubating certain lymphocytes of the spleen in IL_2 gives rise to cells that are not toxic to normal cells but are specifically cytotoxic to certain tumor cells regardless of their natural killer susceptibility. These cells are called lymphokine activating killer (LAK) cells (59). Recent availability of large amounts of recombinant IL_2 has made it possible to evaluate the antitumor activity of this lymphokine in vivo. In animal tumor models it was found that only the combination of transfused LAK cells and repetitive injections of IL_2 resulted in an effective response (92;106). Recently, combined therapy of LAK cells and IL_2 have shown to produce responses in patients with melanoma, renal, colon, and lung cancer (140). However , the treatment is still limited by the potential severity of toxic reactions. IL_2 is being produced on a large scale by several companies.

Tumor necrosis factor (TNF) is a substance thought to be produced by activated macrophages (17). TNF is able to elicit antitumor activity in recipient animals, and shows in-vitro cytotoxic activity against various tumor cell lines. Recently, the gene encoding human TNF has been cloned and expressed in E.coli in several laboratories. This resulted in a worldwide interest in the clinical application of recombinant TNF (128;157). In addition, sera containing TNF have been reported to protect against various organisms, including certain species of malaria parasites (61;159).

Anti human thymocyte globulin (ATG) is a highly immunosuppressive agent prepared from serum obtained from animals immunized with human thymocytes (lymphocytes originating in the thymus). The immunosuppressive activity of ATG was demonstrated many years ago in monkeys, but its clinical use was only established about 1981. Among the factors that played a role in the contradictory results of the various clinical trials are the different immunosuppressive and toxic activities attributed to ATG preparations from different origins. In the RIVM a rabbit ATG was developed which proved to be superior to the various horse ATG's which are commercially available. This rabbit ATG is highly effective in the treatment of acute rejections of kidney transplants obtained from dead donors. In comparison with the conventional treatment with prednisone, a 20 percent increase of graft survival is obtained one year after transplantation. This results in a significant reduction in health care costs. The product is also used in patients with bone marrow dysfunctioning (aplastic anemia) and the treatment of rejections after heart transplantations. Recent observations show that a combination with cyclosporin A leads to the most successful treatment regime.

Recently a new generation of anti lymphocyte antibodies has been described. Monoclonal anti human lymphocyte globulin appears to be active in the treatment of kidney transplant rejection. The advantage of monoclonal anti lymphocyte antibodies, in comparison with the polyclonal rabbit ATG, is that the product is better characterized, standardized, and easier to produce. A more specific modulation of the immune system can be induced. On the other hand, most most side effects, which are inherent to the mechanism of ATG, such as fever, shivering, and sensitization, are also observed after treatment with monoclonal antibodies. A special problem with monoclonal anti lymphocyte antibodies is caused by their high specificity. Some do not cross-react with monkey lymphocytes, which makes preclinical in vivo examination for immunosuppressive activity in monkeys impossible.

Clinical investigations with monoclonal antibodies developed in the RIVM will be done in 1987.

APPENDIX B METHOD OF THE STUDY

The need for examining future health care technology was recognized by the Dutch Steering Committee on Future Health Scenarios (STG) in 1984. (The STG is an independent advisory group to the Dutch government set up in 1983 to carry out scenario studies as an aid to long-term health planning). The STG initiated the Project on Future Health Care Technology. The World Health Organization, European Office (EURO), agreed to support the project financially and logistically.

The project had two specific objectives:
1. To identify future technological developments in health care, with brief descriptions of potential technologies; and
2. To carry out prospective assessments of four high priority technologies or areas of technological development.

The project began in April 1985. A Commission on Future Health Care Technology made up of 10 members and 5 official observers was appointed to guide the project. Surveys of experts were carried out in the United States and Europe. The information from the surveys, supplemented by material from the scientific literature and from interviews, was the basis for the overall descriptions of health care technology. The assistance of these many individuals and groups is specifically acknowledged in appendixes to Volumes I and II of this report.

The project plan called for four technologies to be prospectively assessed. In September 1985, the Commission met and endorsed four cases:
1. implications of neurosciences;
2. biotechnology - probably examining both monoclonal antibodies and vaccines;
3. laser applications, especially in surgery and in the treatment of vascular disease, especially coronary artery disease; and
4. genetic and diagnosis and screening.

Later, with funding from the Ministry of Economic Affairs, medical imaging and home care technology were also developed as case studies.

A detailed description of methods for the entire project is presented in an appendix to Volume I of the report. An updated version may be found in Volume II. And each case study contains a methods description specific to that case.

Late in 1985, a contract was let with CIVI for a report on monoclonal antibodies. The report from the contract was received in 1986 and formed a basis of work on that case study. Using this report and the earlier position paper, dicussions were held with a variety of experts, including officials of RIVM.

The vaccine case was developed at the same time, based on the early draft paper, discussions with experts, literature, and special assistance from RIVM staff. On 20 June 1986, Dr. R. Widdus from the U.S. Institute of Medicine visited the RIVM and the Health Council and discussed the case with project staff.

Work on other case studies prevented intensive work on this case until later in 1986. Nonetheless, material was collected and analyzed.

Early in 1987, the Commission discussed this case and decided that it should focus on vaccines. The issue of monoclonal antibodies had been much publicized. Based on this decision, an approach was made to RIVM to solicit its cooperation. RIVM endorsed the plan to focus on the Dutch situation with vaccines.

During February, March, and April, the report was drafted. RIVM also furnished material, mostly on vaccines.

On 7 May 1987, the Commission on Health Biotechnology of the Health Council reviewed the draft. The Commission gave a number of helpful suggestions. These suggestions were incorporated into the draft report. The Commission reviewed the report at its meeting of 18 May 1987. At that time, some information was still lacking in the report, but was due from the RIVM. The Commission made a few suggestions for changes and agreed to approve the report by mail ballot when it was completed. The report was completed during the next few days, and was transmitted to the Commission in early June. The Commission approved the report, and it was transmitted to the STG in early July.

APPENDIX C GLOSSARY OF TERMS

Acute: In health care, used to describe a condition that has a sudden onset, sharp rise, and short course. Acute diseases are generally completely resolved (compare **Chronic**).

Adjuvant: Material which increases the response to an antigen given at the same time, this probably by improving and prolonging the antigen presentation.

Aerosol: a liquid agent or solution dispersed in the air as a fine mist.

AIDS (acquired immunodeficiency syndrome): A disease believed to be caused by the retrovirus HTLV-III (human T-cell lymphotropic virus, type III) and characterized by a deficiency of the immune system. The primary defect in AIDS is an acquired, persistent, quantitative functional depression of certain white blood cells. This depression often leads to infections caused by micro-organisms and parasites that usually do not produce infections in individuals with normal immunity or to the development of a rare type of cancer (Kaposi's sarcoma).

Allergy: The hypersensitivity of the body cells to a specific substance (antigen, allergen) which results in an antigen-antibody reaction.

Amino acid: An organic acid containing the amino group NH_2; esp: any of the alpha-amino acids that are the chief components of proteins.

Amniocentesis: A procedure that involves withdrawing a sample (usually 2 to 8 ml) of the amniotic fluid surrounding the fetus in utero. The fluid taken contains cells shed by the developing fetus. These can be grown in cell culture and analyzed to detect a variety (over 100) of hereditary diseases. The fluid can also be analyzed for serological or biochemical abnormalities to diagnose or confirm the presence of a developmental disorder.

Angina pectoris: Severe constricting pain in the chest radiating from the region of the heart to the left shoulder and down the arm, accompanied by cardiac oppression due to ischemia. Usually caused by coronary disease.

Antihelmintic: Having the power to destroy or expel intestinal worms.
Anthrax: Disease resulting from infection with Baccillus anthracis. The disease is marked by hemorrhage and serous effusions in the organs and cavities.

Antibiotic: A chemical substance (often produced by a micro-organism) that is administered to fight infections, usually bacterial infections, in humans or animals. The action of the antibiotic is to kill or inhibit the growth of the bacteria. Examples are pencillin, tetracycline, and erythromycin.

Antibody: A blood protein (immunoglobulin) produced by white blood cells in response to the introduction of a specific antigen (usually a protein). Once produced, the antibody has the ability to combine with the specific antigen that stimulated antibody production. This reaction to foreign substances is part of the immune response. See also **Immunoglobulin**.

Antigen: A substance, usually a protein or complex carbohydrate, which, when introduced into the body of a human or other animal, stimulates the production of an antibody that reacts specifically with it.

Anti-idiotype vaccine: Vaccines consisting of anti-idiotype antibodies. These antibodies have structural elements that are not only closely related to the original antigen, but also recognized as such.

Antitoxin: A substance in the serum that binds and neutralizes a toxin, such as that produced by a microorganism. Antitoxin can also be produced in animals such as horses by the injection of gradually increasing doses of toxin. The antitoxin-rich serum can then be withdrawn and used in the treatment of certain human diseases (e.g. rabies, tetanus).

Arthritis: Inflammation of a joint

Attenuated: Weakened, a pathogenic microorganism with reduced virulence.

Auto-immune disease: A disease caused by one's own antibodies

Bacteriology: The scientific study of bacteria.

Bacterium (pl. bacteria): A unicellar vegetable microorganism.

Bacteriuria: The passage of bacteria in the urine.

Basic research: An activity whose aim is to understand vital processes. Basic research has as goal to develope knowledge or understanding. Application of the knowledge occurs through applied research.

BCG: Abbreviation for Bacillus Calmette-Guerin. A descendant of the tubercle bacillus (the causative organism for tuberculosis) that has lost its virulence, used as a vaccine against tuberculosis.

Biochemical: Relating to the chemistry of living organisms and of the changes occurring therein.

Biologics: Medicinal preparations made from living organisms and their products, including serums, vaccines, antigens, and antitoxins.

Bioprocess: Any process that uses complete living cells or their components (e.g., enzymes, chloroplasts) to effect desired physical or chemical changes.

Biosensor: An instrument to detect and measure certain biological materials that is implanted in the human body.

Biotechnology: Techniques that use living organisms or substances from organisms to make or modify a product. 'New' biotechnology refers to recombinant DNA techniques and other sophisticated tools relying on the ability to harness and manipulate genetic material.

Blood: A liquid (plasma) containing red blood cells (erythrocytes), white blood cells (leukocytes), and platelets (thrombocytes) that circulates through the heart, arteries, capillaries, and veins, carrying oxygen and nutrients to body tissues, removing carbon dioxide and other wastes, transferring hormonal messages between organs, preventing bleeding, and transporting antibodies and infection fighting cells to sites of infection.

Blood cells: Erythrocytes (red blood cells), leukocytes (white blood cells), or thrombocytes (platelets).

Bone marrow: The soft fatty substance filling the cavities of long bones.

Cancer: A tumor, the natural course of which is usually fatal. Cancers are divided into two broad categories, carcinoma and sarcoma.

Candida: A type of fungus. Candida albicans often is the cause of pneumonia and meningitis.

Carbohydrate: Anyof various various neutral compounds of carbon, hydrogen, and oxygen (as sugars, starches, and celluloses) most of which are formed by green plants.

Carcinoma: See **Cancer**.

Central nervous system: The brain and spinal cord. The nerves and ganglia outside of the central nervous system constitute the peripheral nervous system.

Chemotherapy: The use of specific chemical agents to arrest the progress of, or eradicate, disease in the body.

Chlamydia: Single-celled organisms that are common in fresh water and damp soil and often are parasitic.

Cholera: An acute epidemic infectious disease which is marked clinically by profuse watery diarrhea, muscular cramps, vomiting and collapse.

Chorionic villus sampling: A technique of antenatal diagnosis by which a sample of tissue is taken from the placenta (whose cells are of fetal origin) and analyzed for the presence or absence of certain heriditary defects.

Chronic: Lingering, lasting, as opposed to acute. A term used to describe persistent or irreversible disease.

Cirrhosis: A degeneration or atrophy of specific cells of any organ with hypertrophy of connective tissue.

Clinical trial: An experiment carried out for the purpose of evaluating the efficacy and safety of a health care technology. The nature of the control group is a critical issue in a clinical trial. See **Control group**, **Randomized clinical trial**.

Clone: A group of cells that have arisen from a single cell as a result of asexual reproduction.

Communicable disease: transmittable disease.

Complement: The thermolabile substance in normal blood serum and plasma that in combination with antibodies causes the destruction of bacteria, foreign blood corpuscles, and other antigens.

Congenital: Existing at birth.

Congenital abnormality: Any abnormality in structure or function, whether genetic or not, that has a prenatal origin (is present at birth). Congenital abnormalities can be genetic, chromosomal, or caused by endogenous or exogenous agents. Some prefer the term **Developmental disorder.**

Contamination: Pollution, soiling with infectious matter.

Control group: In a randomized clinical trial, the group receiving no treatment or some treatment with which the group receiving experimental treatment is compared. The control treatment is generally a standard treatment, a placebo, or no treatment. Compare **Experimental group.**

Controlled clinical trial: See **Clinical trial.**

Convulsion: A violent involuntary muscular contraction.

Cost-benefit analysis (CBA): An analytical technique that compares the costs of a project or technological application to the resultant benefits, with both costs and benefits expressed by the same measure. This measure is nearly always monetary.

Cost-effectiveness analysis (CEA): An analytical technique that compares the costs of a project or of alternative projects to the resultant benefits, with costs and benefits/effectiveness expressed by different measures. Costs are usually expressed in dollars, but benefits/effectiveness are ordinarily expressed in terms such as 'lives saved,' 'disability avoided,' 'quality-adjusted life years saved,' or any other relevant objectives.

Cystic fibrosis: A heriditary disorder characterized by widespread dysfunction of glands. Breathing problems and pulmonary infection are characteristic of the disease.

Cytomegalovirus: A virus causing infection of the fetus in utero, with associated irreversible damage to the central nervous system.

Cytotoxin: A substance (as a toxin or antibody) having toxic effects on cells.

Development: See **Applied research.** Also **Targeted development.**

Developmental disorder: See Congenital abnormality.

Diphtheria: An infectious disease due to the Corynebacterium diphteriae baccillus, marked by inflammation of the nose or throat, and by more or less pronounced symptoms of toxemia.

Disability: A term used to denote the presence of one or more functional limitations. A person with a disability has a limited ability or an inability to perform one or more basic life functions (e.g., walking) at a level considered 'typical.' Compare to **Handicap.**

DNA: Deoxyribonucleic acid. The nucleic acid in chromosomes that codes for the genetic information. See also **Gene.**

DNA probe: A sequence of DNA that is used to detect the presence of a particular nucleotide base sequence. See **Probe.**

Down's syndrome: A disorder caused by a specific abnormality of one chromosome. Down syndrome is characterized by mental retardation and may also include congenital heart defects, immune system abnormalities, various morphological abnormalities and a reduced life expectancy. It has been shown to increase in frequency with advanced maternal age.

Duchenne muscular dystrophy: Progressive wasting (atrophy) of the muscles beginning in the arms. It is a genetic disease with its onset in early childhood, almost always in males. Those with the disease seldom survive to adulthood.

Effectiveness: Same as efficacy (see below) except that it refers to '...average or actual conditions of use.'

Efficacy: The probability of benefit to individuals in a defined population from a medical technology applied for a given medical problem under ideal conditions of use.

Electrophoresis: A technique for separating different molecules based on their differential movement in an electric field. The differential movement is a complex function of molecule size, shape, and net electrical charge.

Embolism: Obstruction or occlusion of a vessel by a transported clot.

Endocrine: Refers to a gland that furnishes an internal secretion. Examples are the pancreas and the gonads.

Endogenous: Developing or originating within the organism, or arising from causes within the organism.

Enzyme: Any of a group of proteins that are produced by living cells and that mediate and promote the chemical processes of life without themselves being altered or destroyed.

Epidemiology: The scientific study of the distribution and determinants of diseases and health conditions in population groups.

Epitope: Segment of an antigen provoking a reaction by the immune system.

Etiology: Cause or origin.

Experimental group: In a randomized clinical trial, the group receiving the treatment being evaluated for safety and efficacy. The experimental treatment may be a new technology, an existing technology applied to a new problem, or an accepted treatment about whose safety or efficacy there is doubt. Compare **Control group**.

False negative: A negative test esult in an individual who actually does have the disease of characteristic being tested for. The person is incorrectly diagnosed as not having a particular disease or characteristic.

False positive: A positive test result in an individual who does not have the disease or characteristic being tested for. I.e., the individual is incorrectly diagnosed as having a particular disease or characteristic.

Fermentation: A chemical change induced by a chemical or living ferment in a complex organic compound whereby the substance is split up into more simple compounds.

Fetus: The unborn from the end of the third month to the moment of birth.

Fibrin: An elastic filamentous protein formed in the coagulation of blood.

Fluorescent: Possessing the quality of becoming self-luminous when exposed to light or to other rays.

Gamma globulin: A group of plasma proteins that have antibody activity and which in concentrated form may be used for passive immunization against a number of diseases and in the treatment of gamma globulin deficiency. Also called 'immune globulins.'

Gene: The portion of a DNA molecule that comprises the basic functional unit of heredity; a sequence of DNA that produces a specific product.

Gene therapy: See **Genetic engineering**.

Genetic: Inherited. Carried in the genes.

Genetic engineering: Active manipulation of the genetic material for some purpose, such as removing harmful genes or improving certain genetic traits in animals.

Germ cell: An egg or sperm or one of their antecedent cells.

Glaucoma: The increase of the fluids of the eyeball, raising intraocular pressure.

Glycolipid: A lipid that contains a carbohydrate

Gonorrhea: An inflammation of the mucous membrane of the genital tract induced by gonococcus. The disease is transferred by sexual intercourse.

Handicap: Inability to perform one or more life functions (e.g., eating, conversing, working) at a 'typical' level, caused by the interaction of an individual's disability with the physical and social environments in which that person is functioning or expected to function. Compare to **Disability**.

Health care technology: The drugs, devices, and medical and surgical procedures used in medical care, and the organizational and support systems within which such care is provided.

Hemoglobin: The coloring matter of the blood. It is a protein in combination with an iron compound whose function is to carry oxygen and carbon dioxide.

Hemophilia: A rare, hereditary bleeding disorder distinguished by a deficiency of one or more coagulation factors, e.g. factor VIII (hemophilia A). Hemophilia is most often seen in males, and most often transmitted to offspring by asymptomatic females.

Hemophilus influenzae: A bacterium that causes disease of the upper respiratory tract and the bronchopulmonary tree (bronchi and lungs).

Hepatitis: Inflammation of the liver which may be due any of several causes (including viruses).

Hepatitis A: Viral hepatitis, type A. An acute illness caused by hepatitis A virus occurring mostly in children and young adults. It is usually transmitted by oral ingestion of contaminated matter, though it may also be transmitted parenterally (by contaminated needles or administration of blood products). Formerly known as 'infectious hepatitis.'

Hepatitis B: Viral hepatitis, type B. An acute illness caused by hepatitis B virus. It was formerly thought to be transmitted only through parenteral exposure (contaminated needles or administration of blood products), but is now known also to be transmitted by oral ingestion of contaminated matter. Formerly known as 'serum hepatitis.'

Heriditary: Inherited. See **Gene**.

Herpes genitalis: Herpes simplex of the penis or vulva.

Hormone: A chemical substance released into the circulatory system by glands belonging to the endocrine system, and that has a specific regulatory effect on another organ; functions regulated include metabolism, growth, and the development of secondary sex characteristics.

Huntington's disease: A rare genetic disease characterized by chronic progressive disorders of movement and mental deterioration culminating in dementia. The disease is transmitted as an autosomal dominant trait, but usually does not manifest itself until a person is between the ages of 30 and 50. Death usually results within 15 years. Also called 'Huntington's chorea.'

Hybridoma: Long-lived cells, produced by fusion of an antibody-forming cell such as a lymphocyte with a tumor cell such as a mouse myeloma cell.

Hypopituitarism: A condition due to diminished activity of the hypophysis of the pituitary gland.

Idiotype: Part of an antibody that recognizes the antigen.

Immune: Protected against disease by innate or acquired (active or passive) immunity.

Immune deficiency disease: A disease characterized by the inability to make sufficient quantities of normal antibody. It can be treated by the injection of immunoglobulin.

Immune globulin: See **Immunoglobulin.**

Immune response: The reaction of an organism after exposure to certain foreign substances (antigens). Immune responses are often highly complex, and may involve the production of immunoglobulins (antibodies) from special cells (lymphocytes), as well as a varying set of physical and chemical responses from other cells of the immune system. The immune response is often referred to as being either humoral (by antibodies in the blood serum), cellular (by white blood cells), or both.

Immune system: Specialized groups of body cells and cell products that respond to foreign organisms and substances in the body. The cell products are largely immunoglobulins (antibodies), produced by specialized white blood cells known as lymphocytes. Some lymphocytes and various other cells of the immune system directly attack foreign organisms or mediate this attack.

Immunity: The condition of being immune; an organism's capacity to resist a particular disease. Immunity may be either innate or acquired. Innate immunity is natural or inherited. Acquired immunity may be active (resulting from either previous exposure to the disease-causing agent or vaccination) or passive (resulting from the transfer of preformed antibodies by immune serum or from mother to fetus).

Immunization: The deliberate introduction of an antigenic substance (vaccination, or active immunization) or antibodies (passive immunization) into an individual, to produce immunity to a disease. Compare **Vaccination.**

Immunoassay: The use of antibodies to identify and quantify antigenic substances. The binding of antibodies to antigen is often accompanied by tracers such as radioisotopes.

Immunoglobulin: A plasma protein of animal origin endowed with known antibody activity. Immunoglobulins function as specific antibodies and are responsible for certain aspects of immunity. They are found in the serum, in other body fluids, and in tissues. Immunoglobulin is the key feature of B cells, through which they recognize specific antigens.

Immunology: The scientific study of immunity, induced sensitivity, and allergy.

Immunosuppression: Suppression of natural immune responces.

Immunotherapy: Treatment of or prophylaxis against disease by means of antigens or antigenic preparations.

Incidence: The frequency of new occurrences of disease within a defined time interval. Incidence rate is the number of new cases of specified disease over a specified period of time, usually 1 year, divided by the number of people in a population. Compare **Prevalence**.

Infarction: Obstruction of local blood circulation leading to an area of necrosis.

Infection: The invasion and proliferation of any pathogenic organism in body tissues.

Innovation: A new device, product, or process introduced to practice for the first time. Innovations are valued for their capacity to improve the quality or decrease the costs of a given process or product. Also, something perceived to be new. In addition, innovation is widely used to refer to the process by which technological change occurs.

Insulin: A hormone secreted by the isles of Langerhans that is essential esp. for the metabolism of carbohydrates.

Interferon: A family of proteins produced rapidly by many cells in response to virus infection, which block the replication of viruses in other cells.

Intravenous: Within a vein.

In vitro: Literally, 'in glass,' pertaining to a biological process or reaction taking place in an artificial environment, usually a laboratory. Sometimes used to include the growth of cells from multicellular organisms under cell culture conditions.

In vivo: Literally, 'in the living,' pertaining to a biological process or reaction taking place in a living cell or organism.

Lesion: Structural change in an organ. See **Pathology**.

Leukemia: A disease of the blood characterized by a persistent increase in the number of white blood cells and associated with changes in the spleen, bone marrow, and lymphoid system.

Leukocyte: Any of the white or colorless nucleated cells that occur in blood.

Lipid: Any of the various substances that are soluble in nonpolar organic solvents (as chloroform and ether), that with proteins and carbohydrates constitute teh principle structural components of living cells, and that include fats, waxes, and related and derivated compounds.

Liposome: A structure with a lipid membrane like that of a cell which can be filled with specific substances and then used as a delivery vehicle transporting those substances to the interior of a targeted cell by fusion with the cell's own membrane.

Lymph gland (or lymph node): One of the rounded masses of lymphoid tissue. They contain numerous cells that, when carried of by the flow of lymph through the node, become lymphocytes.

Lymphocyte: A small cell found in blood and the lymph, 'policing' the body for non-self material (antigens).

Lymphoma: A tumor of lymphoid tissue

Lymphokines: Lymphocyte products affecting macrophages and other cells.

Lysis: Irreversible leakage of cell contents following membrane damage.

Lytic agent: A substance causing lysis.

Macrophage: A large tissue cell responsible for removing damaged cells, bacteria, etc..

Malaria: A disease that is caused by sporozoan parasites in the red blood cells, is transmitted by the bite of certain mosquitoes, and is characterized by periodic attacks of chills and fever.

Malignant: Resistant to treatment; tending to grow worse.

Medical technology: See **Health care technology**.

Meningitis: Inflammation of the membranes of the brain or spinal cord.

Metabolic: Referring to metabolism.

Metabolism: The sum of the chemical changes that make up the process of nutrition of the organism.

Metabolite: A product of metabolism

Metastasis: The shifting of a disease, or its local manifestations, from one part of the body to another. In cancer, the appearance of neoplasms in parts of the body remote from the seat of the primary tumor.

Microbial: Relating to a microorganism

Microbiology: The science or study of microorganisms.

Microorganism: A minute, microscopic or submicroscopic living organism. Examples are bacteria, mycoplasma, viruses, and protozoa.

Molecule: The smallest possible quantity of a substance that can exist independently and still retain the properties of the substance of which it forms a part. It is formed by a combination of two or more atoms.

Molecular biology: The study of biology at the level of individual molecules, such as proteins and DNA.

Monoclonal antibodies (MAbs): Antibodies derived from a single source or clone of cell. MAbs recognize only one type of antigen.

Morbidity: The condition of being diseased. The morbidity rate is the ratio of sick to well persons in a community.

Mortality rate: The death rate, often made explicit for a particular characteristic, e.g., age, sex, or specific cause of death. A mortality rate contains three essential elements: 1) the number of people in a population group exposed to the risk of death; 2) a time factor; 3) the number of deaths occurring in the exposed population during a certain time period.

Mucosal immunity: Immunity to infection of the mucous membranes (of the mouth, vagina, etc.). See **Immunity**.

Mucous: Relating to a membrane secreting mucus, which lines passages and cavities communicating with the exterior.

Mutagenesis: The production of a mutation (change in genetic information).

Myasthenia gravis: A chronic progressive muscular weakness, usually beginning in the face and throat.

Mycoplasma: Microorganisms without cell walls that are intermediate in some respects between viruses and bacteria and are mostly parasitic usually in mamals.

Myocardial: Relating to the heart muscle.

Myocardial infarction: Infarction of the heart muscle.

Neurological: Referring to the nervous system (including the brain).

Nuclear magnetic resonance spectoscopy:

Nucleic acid: Any of various acids composed of a sugar or derivate of a sugar, phosphoric acid, and a base and found especially in cel nuclei.

Oligosaccharide: A saccharide that contains a known small number of mono-saccharide units.

Oncogenes: Genes associated with cancer formation.

Osteoporosis: A disease of bone marked by loss of calcium and resulting softened or brittle bone, prone to fractures. It occurs frequently in elderly people, particularly women.

Pancreas: A gland that secretes digestive enzymes and the hormone insulin.

Parasite: An organism living in or on another organisms obtaining benefits from the host which it usually injures.

Parenteral: Throughout the body. Usually refers to administration by injection.

Pathogenesis: The mode of origin or development of any disease.

Pathogenic: Causing disease.

Pathological: Relating to pathology. Morbid or diseased.

Pathologist: One who interprets and diagnoses the changes caused by disease in tissues.

Pathology: The scientific study of the essential nature of disease and of the associated structural and functional changes in tissues and organs that are the result of disease. The field of pathology often deals with the diagnosis of disease. The term is also frequently used as a synonym for 'disease.'

Peptide: A combination of two or more aminoacids (a type of organic acid). A protein, in contrast, is a long chain of aminoacides. See **Protein**.

Peridontal: Surrouding a tooth or part of a tooth.

Perinatal: Around the time of birth.

Phagocytosis: Engulfment of a particle by a cell. The great majority of foreign materials entering the tissues are ultimately disposed of by this mechanism.

Pharmacology: The branch of science that is concerned with drugs (pharmaceuticals).

Phenylketonuria: An inherited disease of metabolism, which can result in mental retardation, spasticity, slow physical development, speech difficulties, and so forth. The name comes from the fact that phenylketones (certain chemicals) are found in the urine. Mass screening programs have made early treatment possible, and few people with the disease develop such problems today in industrialized countries.

Plasma: The liquid portion of the blood in which particulate components of the blood are suspended. See **Serum**..

Plasmid: A cellular element that exists and replicates autonomously in the cytoplasm.

Poliomyelitis: An acute infectious virus disease characterized by fever, motor paralysis, and atrophy of skeletal muscles often with permanent disability and deformity and marked by inflammation of nerve cells in the spinal cord.

Polypeptide: A peptide of three or more amino acids (See **Protein**, **Peptide**).

Polysaccharide: A complex carbohydrate (as sugars, cellulose, starch, or glycogen)

Postnatal: Occurring after birth.

Prenatal: Occurring or formed before birth. Also called 'antenatal.'

Prevalence: The total number of cases of disease, infected persons, or persons with disabilities or some other condition, in existence in a particular area or population at a certain time. The prevalence rate is the total number (prevalence) in relation to the size of the population. Compare **Incidence**.

Probe: Any biochemical substance tagged or labelled with a tracer substance (a radioactive isotope or specific dye-absorbing compound) and used to locate or identify a specific gene or gene product.

Protein: A polypeptide consisting of amino acids. In their biologically active states, they function as structural elements of cells and tissues or as catalysts in metabolism (enzymes).

Protozoa: Animals consisting of a single cell or of an aggregation of non-differentiated cells.

Pyuria: Urinary tract infection

Rabies: An acute infectious disease characterized by spasm of the muscles of respiration, madness, and other symptoms of profound disturbance of the central nervous system.

Radioactive: The property possessed by some elements of spontaneously emitting alpha or beta rays and sometimes gamma rays by the desintegration of the nuclei of atoms.

Randomized clinical trial (RCT): An experiment designed to test the safety and efficacy of a medical technology in which people are randomly allocated to experimental or control groups, and outcomes are compared.

Receptor: A molecular grouping on the cell surface that can bind other specific molecules, such as hormones, neurotransmitters, and antigens. After the binding, the activity of the cell is affected in a specific way.

Recombinant DNA technology: The technique developed in the 1970's that allows genes to be combined or 'spliced.' The most common application so far has been to insert new genes into bacterial cells to give the bacterium abilities it did not previously have. Recombinant DNA technology has not yet been used in humans, but it is the basis for human gene therapy, which may begin soon.

Red blood cells: The cells in the blood that contain hemoglobin and carry oxygen and carbon dioxide. Also called erythrocytes.

Risk: A measure of the probability of an adverse or untoward outcome and the severity of the resultant harm to health of individuals in a defined population and associated with the use of a medical technology applied for a given medical problem under specified conditions of use.

RNA (ribonucleic acid): The nucleic acid found mainly in the nucleolus and ribosomes of the cell and associated with the control of cellular chemical activities.

Rota virus: A specific small virus. It causes, for example, a bacterial gastro-enteritis in small children.

Rubella: German measles. A viral disease of childhood, usually mild. However, when pregnant women acquire the disease, it can have serious consequences for the fetus.

Safety: A judgment of the acceptability of risk in a specified situation. See also **Risk**.

Schistosomiasis: Infestation with a species of Schistosoma, comprising the bloodflukes, in which the sexes are distinct. Their eggs invade tract walls, causing severe irritation and inflammation of those parts.

Screening: An attempt to detect high risk individuals or those with disorders that have not yet caused symptoms. Screening is followed by specific diagnostic procedures when positive. It is done for the purpose of intervention, i.e., to cure the disease or prevent problems associated with it.

Sensitivity: The true positive ratio. In referring to a diagnostic test, it is the extent to which abnormals are correctly classified.

Serological: Related to serology

Serology: The branch of science dealing with serum, especially with specific immune serum.

Serum: The fluid portion of the blood obtained after the blood has coagulated. See **Plasma**.

Sickle cell disease: A hereditary disease caused by the presence of a defective hemoglobin. Patients with sickle-cell disease have red blood cells that tend to deform into a sickle-like shape when the abnormal hemoglobin crystallizes. The specific defect is caused by an abnormal gene. Also called 'sickle-cell anemia.' There is currently no effective treatment.

Slow virus: A virus whose disease only appears some time (i.e., years) later.

Somatostatin: A growth hormone inhibiting factor produced by the hypothalamus (part of the brain) the pancreas and the gastro-intestinal tract.

Somatic: A term used to refer to body tissues apart from reproductive (germinal) tissues.

Specificity: The true negative ratio. In referring to a diagnostic test, it is the extent to which normals are correctly classified. Compare **sensitivity**.

Spleen: A highly vascular organ concerned with final destruction of blood cells, storage of blood, and production of lymphocytes.

Streptococcus: A genus of the tribe Streptococcae, consisting of rod-like organisms occuring in pairs or large chains.

Subunit vaccine: A vaccine that contains only portions of an antigenic molecule from a pathogen. Subunit vaccines can be prepared by using recombinant DNA technology to produce all or part of the antigenic molecule or by artificial (chemical) synthesis of short peptides.

Suspension: The diffusion through a liquid of a solid in finely divided particles.

Synthetic vaccine: Vaccines containing peptides or oligosaccharides mimicking specific sites on the surface of a antigen.

Targeted development: The product-oriented development of a technology after basic and applied research have accumulated sufficient knowledge and technical means to make final realization of the envisaged produce rather likely.

Technology: The application of organized knowledge to practical ends.

Technology assessment: In general, a comprehensive form of policy research that examines the technical, economic, and social consequences of technological applications. It is especially concerned with unintended, indirect, or delayed social impacts. In health policy, however, the term more often is used to mean any form of policy analysis concerned with health care technology, especially the evaluation of efficacy and safety.

Technology diffusion: The diffusion or spread of a medical technology into the health care system. It is generally thought to involve two phases: the initial phase in which decisions are made to adopt or reject the technology, and a subsequent phase in which decisions are made to use the technology.

Tetanus: An infectious disease marked by painful tonic muscular contractions; it is caused by the toxin of Bacillus tetani acting upon the central nervous system.

Thalassaemia: A group of autosomal recessive genetic disorders characterized by abnormalities in hemoglobin that lead to an overall deficiency of adult hemoglobin. The thalassaemias are most common in people of Mediterranean, Middle Eastern, and Asian descent.

Thrombus (pl. thrombi): A solid mass of fibrin, platelets, and in most instances erythrocytes, in a blood vessel.

Toxin: A poisonous substance that is a specific product of the metabolic activities of a living organism. It is typically capable of inducing antibody formation.

Toxoid: A toxin of a pathogenic organism treated so as to destroy its toxicity but leave it capable of inducing the formation of antibodies on injection.

Toxoplasmosis: Infection with the protozoan parasite Toxoplasma. The species **Toxoplasma gondii** can cause acute encephalitis in children.

Typhoid fever: A communicable disease caused by bacteria and marked especially by fever, diarrhea, prostration, headache, and intestinal inflammation.

Upper respiratory infection: An infection of the upper parts of the respiratory system, especially the nose and throat, often called a 'cold'.

Vaccination: The deliberate introduction of an antigenic substance (vaccine) into an individual, with the aim of producing active immunity to a disease. Compare **Immunization**.

Vaccine: A preparation of living, attenuated, or killed bacteria or viruses, fractions thereof, or synthesized antigens identical or similar to those found in the disease-causing organisms, administered to produce or increase immunity to a particular disease.

Varicella zoster: The virus causing chickenpox.

Venous: Related to the veins, blood vessels that return blood to the heart.

Virus: Any of a large group of submicroscopic agents infecting plants, animals, and bacteria and characterized by a total dependence on living cells for reproduction and metabolism.

Vitamins: A group of compounds unrelated to each other, present in minute amounts in natural foods. They are essential to normal metabolism and their lack causes certain diseases.

White blood cells: The cells in the blood that constitute part of the immune system. They are divided into two main types, lymphocytes and granulocytes. White blood cells are also known as leucocytes.

Yeast: A ferment consisting of a culture of Saccharomyces (cerevisiae).

APPENDIX D REFERENCES

1. van Aken WG. Bloedtechnologie. In Toekomstverkenningen. Jaarboek Gezondheidsraad 1986. The Hague, The Netherlands: 167-174.

2. Albritton R. Cost-benefits of measles eradication: effects of a federal intervention. Policy Analysis 1978; pp. 1-21.

3. Alter HJ. The evolution, implications, and applications of the hepatitis B vaccine (editorial). JAMA 1982; 247: 2272-2275.

4. Audibert F. Synthetic adjuvants and synthetic vaccines. Vaccine 1985; 3: 155-156.

5. Axnick N, Shavell S, Witte J. Benefits due to immunization against measles. Public Health Reports 1969; 84: 673-680.

6. Banta HD, Behney CJ, Willems JS. Toward rational technology in medicine. New York: Springer Publishing Company, 1981.

7. Barin F, Goudeau A, Brechot C, et al. Further studies on production and characterization of HBsAg derived from a human hepatoma cell line (PLC/PRF/5). In Papaevangelou G, Hennessen W eds. Viral hepatitis: standardization in immunoprophylaxis of infections by hepatitis viruses. Developments in Biological Standards 1983;54: 81-92.

8. Barre-Sinoussi F, Chermann J, Rey F, et al. Isolation of a T-lymphotropic retrovirus from a patient at risk for acquired immuno deficiency syndrome. Science 1983; 220: 868-871.

9. Beale AJ. Hybrid vaccinia virus for mass hepatitis immunization? Nature 1983; 302: 476-477.

10. Beale J. Recombinant vaccinia for prevention of hepatitis B. Nature 1984; 311: 12-13.

11. Beale J. Synthetic peptides as the basis for future vaccines. Nature 1982; 298: 14-15.

12. Beardsly T. WHO back to vector vaccines. Nature 1984; 312: 299.

13. Beasley RP, Lin C-C, Hwang L-Y, Chien C-S. Hepatocellular carcinoma and hepatitis B virus. Lancet 1981; 2: 1129-1133.

14. Behbehani AM. The smallpox story: life and death of an old disease. Microbiological Reviews 1983; 47: 455-509.

15. Beran GW, Crowley AJ. Toward worldwide rabies control. WHO Chronicle 1983; 37: 192-196.

16. Berman PW, Nunes W, Fennie C, Lasky LA. Expression of recombinant AIDS retrovirus envelope protein analogues in genetically engineered cell lines. Abstracts of the Second International Conference on AIDS, p.15. Paris, June 23-25, 1986.

17. Beutler B, Greenwald D, Hulmes JD, Chang M, Pan CE, Mathison J, Ulevich R, Cerami A. Identity of tumor necrosis factor and macrophage-secreted factor cachectin. Nature 1985; 316: 552-554.

18. Bezold C ed. Pharmaceuticals in the year 2000, the changing context for drug R&D. Alexandria, Virginia: Institute for Alternative Futures, 1983.

19. Bialy H. Biotechnologies converge on new vaccines. Biotechnology, January 1985: 11.

20. Bodde T. Interferon: will it live up to its promise? Bioscience 1982; 32: 13-15.

21. Borst P. Moleculaire biologie. In Toekomstverkenningen. Jaarboek Gezondheidsraad 1986. The Hague, The Netherlands: 141-150

22. Brodie DC, Smith WE. Implications of new technology for pharmacy education and practice. American Journal of Hospital Pharmacy 1985; 42: 81-95.

23. Brummelhuis HGJ, Wilson-De Sturler LA, Raap AK. Preparations of hepatitis B vaccine by heat-inactivation. In Maupas P, Guersy P eds. Hepatitis B vaccine. Amsterdam: Elsevier/North Holland 1981: 51-56.

24. Burg C. The prospects for medicine in the next 20 years. Presented at the Second European Seminar for Leading Public Health Administrators on Health for All by the Year 2000, Oslo, Norway, 24-30 August 1983.

25. Centers for Disease Control. Pertussis surveillance 1979-1981. Morbidity and Mortality Weekly Report 1982; 31: 333-336.

26. Centers for Disease Control. Recommendations of the Immunization

Practices Advisory Committee: prevention and control of influenza. Morbidity and Mortality Weekly Report 1984; 33: 253-260, 265-266.

27. Check WA. New drugs and drug-delivery systems in the year 2000. American Journal of Hospital Pharmacy 1984; 41: 1536-1547.

28. Chin J. The status and challenge of communicable disease control. In Last JM. Public health and preventive medicine. Norwalk, Connecticut: Appleton-Century-Crofts, 1986: 103-107.

29. Clements ML, Tierney EL, Murphy BR. Response of seronegative and seropositive adult volunteers to live attentuated cold-adapted reassortant influenza A virus vaccine. Journal of Clinical Microbiology 1985; 21: 997-999.

30. Cochi S. Quoted in Koplan (1984)

31. Colorado Department of Social Sciences. A study to determine the cost effectiveness of the pneumovax inoculation program implemented by the Colorado Medicaid Program. Denver, 1980.

32. Committee on Science, Engineering, and Public Policy of the National Academy of Sciences, the National Academy of Engineering, and the Institute of Medicine. Outlook of science and technology: the next five years. Volume III. Washington, D.C.: National Academy Press, 1982.

33. Conference Reports. New approaches to vaccine development. Vaccine 1985; 3: 347-348.

34. Congressional Budget Office. Proposed pneumococcal vaccination benefits: their impact on Medicare outlays. Washington, DC, 1980.

35. Corey L, Adams HG, Brown ZA, Holmes KK. Genital herpes simplex virus infection: clinical manifestations, course, and complications. Annals of Internal Medicine 1983; 98: 958-972.

36. Coutinho RA, Lelie N, Albrecht-Van Lent P, Reerink-Bongers EE, Stoutjesdijk L, Dees P, Nivard J, Huisman J, Reesink HW. Efficacy of heat inactivated hepatitis B vaccine in male homosexuals: outcome of a placebo controlled double blind trial. British Medical Journal 1983; 286: 1305-1308.

37. Davenport FM. Influenza viruses. In Evans AS ed. Viral infections of humans. New York: Plenum, 1982: 373-396.

38. Doshi ML. Accuracy of consumer performed in-home tests for early pregnancy detection. American Journal of Public Health 1986; 76: 512-514.

40. Dougan G, Highfield P. Molecular biology, the new genetics and vaccine development. Medical Laboratory Sciences 1985; 42: 393-398.

41. Douglas RG. Herpes simplex virus infections. In Wyngaarden JB, Smith LH eds. Cecil textbook of medicine. Philadelphia: W.B. Saunders Compnay, 1982: 1646-1649.

42. Dreesman GR, Sanchez Y, Ionescu-Matiu I, Sparrow JT, Six HR, Peterson DL, Hollinger FB, Melnick JL. Antibody to hepatitis B surface antigen after a single inoculation of the uncoupled synthetic HBsAg peptides. Nature 1982; 295: 158-160.

43. Drotman DP, Curran JW. Epidemiology and prevention of acquired immunodeficiency syndrome (AIDS). In Last JM. Public health and preventive medicine. Norwalk, Connecticut: Appleton-Century-Crofts, 1986: 459-466.

44. ECRI. Tumor markers. The laboratory's role in cancer patient management. Journal of Health Care Technology 1985; 2: 105-128.

45. Editorial. Gene therapy method shows promise. Science 1985; 223: 1376.

46. Ekblom M, Elo O, Laurinkari J, Niemela P. Costs and benefits of measles vaccination in Finland. Scandinavian Journal of Social Medicine 1978; 6: 111-115.

47. Elo O. Health and economic consequences of rubella. Acta Universitatis Tamperensis, series A 1975; 60: 27-47

48. Farber M, Finkelstein S. A cost-benefit analysis of a mandatory premarital rubella-antibody screening program. The New England Journal of Medicine 1979; 300: 395-400.

49. Fauci A, Macher A, Longo D, et al. Acquired immunodeficiency syndrome: epidemiological, clinical, immunogenic and therapeutic considerations. Annals of Internal Medicine 1984; 100: 92-106.

50. Foege WH. Banishing measles from the world. World Health Forum 1984; 5: 63-65.

51. Fougereau M, Dausset J eds. Immunology 80. Progress in Immunology IV. London: Academic Press, 1980.
52. Francis DP, Essex M, Maynard JE. Feline leukemia virus and hepatitis B virus: a comparison of late manifestations. Progress in Medical Virology. 1981; 27: 127-132.

53. Fudenberg HH. Fiscal returns of biomedical research. The Journal of Investigative Dermatology 1983; 61: 321-329.

54. Gezondheidsraad. Medische biotechnologie. The Hague, The Netherlands. 24 October 1985.

55. Gezondheidsraad. Vaccinatie tegen influenza seizoen 1985-1986. The Hague, The Netherlands. 9 May 1985.

56. Gezondheidsraad. Verslag inzake ongewenste bijwerkingen vaccins rijksvaccinatieprogramma in 1985. The Hague, The Netherlands, 1986.

57. Gilbert W, Bodmer WF. Two cheers for human gene sequencing. The Scientist 1986; 1: 11-12.

58. Goudeau A, Coursaget P, Barin F, et al. Prevention of hepatitis B by active and passive-active immunization. In Szmuness W, Alter HJ, Maynard JE eds. Viral Hepatitis: 1981 International Symposium. Philadelphia: Franklin Institute Press, 1982: 509-525.

59. Grimm EA, Mazumder A, Zhang HZ, Rosenberg SA. Lymphokine-activated killer cell phenomenon. Lysis of natural killer resistant fresh solid tumor cells by interleukin-2 activated autologous human peripheral blood lymphocytes. Journal of Experimental Medicine 1982; 155: 1823-1841.

60. Haaff EO, Dresner SM, Kelley DR, Ratcliff TL, Shapiro A, Catalonal WJ. Role of immunotherapy in the prevention of recurrence and invasion of urothelial bladder tumors: a review. World Journal of Urology 1985; 3: 76-85.

61. Haidaris CG, Haynes JD, Meltzner MS, Allison AC. Serum containing tumor necrosis factor is cytotoxic for the human malaria parasite Plasmodium falciparum. Infectious Immunology 1983; 42: 385-393.

62. Hannik. Discussion. Proceedings of the Fourth International Symposium on Pertussis. Development of Biological Standards 1985; 61: 477-507.

63. Hannik CA, Cohen H. Pertussis vaccine experience in the Netherlands. Bethesda, Maryland: US Department of Health, Education, and Welfare, Public Health Service, National Institutes of Health, 1979: 279-282 (DHEW Publication No. NIH 79-1830).

64. Hanshaw JB. Cytomegalovirus infections. In Wyngaarden JB, Smith LH eds. Cecil textbook of medicine. Philadelphia: W.B. Saunders Company, 1982: 1649-1651.

65. Henderson DA. The eradication of smallpox. In Last JM. Public health and preventive medicine. Norwalk, Connecticut: Appleton-Century-Crofts, 1986: 129-138.

66. Hilleman MR. Newer directions in vaccine development and utilization. The Journal of Infectious Diseases 1985; 151: 407-419.

67. Hilleman MR, Buynak EB, McAleer WJ, et al. Hepatitis B and hepatitis A vaccines. In Szmuness W, Alter HJ, Maynard JE eds. Viral Hepatitis: 1981 International Symposium. Philadelphia: Franklin Institute Press, 1982: 385-397.

68. Hilleman M, Larson VM, Lehman ED, Salerno RA, Conrad PG, McLean AA. Subunit Herpes simplex vaccine. In Nahmias A, Dowdle W, Schinazi R eds. The human herpes viruses. An interdiscipliarry perspective. New York: Elsevier, 1981: 503-506.

69. Hinman AR. Potential candidates for eradiction. World eradiction of measles. Review on Infectious Diseases 1982; 4: 933-999.

70. Hinman AR, Koplan JP. Pertussis and pertussis vaccine: reanalysis of benefits, risks, and costs. Journal of the American Medical Association 1984; 251: 3109-3113.

71. Hodgkin P, Yoxen E. Biotechnology and general practice, recombinant DNA, monoclonal antibodies and genetic probes. Journal of the Royal College of General Practitioners 1985; 35: 484-487.

72. Holtzman NA. The promise and peril of genetic testing. Baltimore, Maryland: The Johns Hopkins University Press (forthcoming).

73. Institute of Medicine. Confronting AIDS: directions for public health, health care, and research. Washington, DC: National Academy Press, 1986.

74. Institute of Medicine. New vaccine development, establishing

priorities. Volume I. Diseases of importance in the United States. Washington, DC: National Academy Press, 1985.

75. Isaacson RE. Development of vaccines for bacterial diseases using recombinant DNA technology. Avian Diseases 1985; 30: 28-36.

76. Jacobs I, Salazar AM, Herndon R, et al. Multicentre double-blind study of effect of intrathecally administered natural human fibroblast interferon on exacerbations of multiple sclerosis. The Lancet 1986; 2: 1411-1414.

77. Johnson JS. Human insulin from recombinant DNA technology. Science 1983; 219: 632-637.

78. Junginger HE. Research in the division of pharmaceutical technology. Pharmaceutisch Weekblad, Scientific Edition 1985; 7: 59-62.

79. Katz S. Whooping cough (Pertussis). In Wyngaarden JB, Smith LH eds. Cecil textbook of medicine. Philadelphia: W.B. Saunders Compnay, 1982: 1487-1490.

80. Kennedy RC, Melnick JL, Dresman GR. Anti-idiotypes and immunity, Scientific American 1986; 255: 40-48.

81. Kieny MP, Rautmann G, Schmitt D, Dott K, Wain-Hobson S, Alizon M, Girard M, Chaumaret S, Laurent A, Montagnier L, Lecocq JP. AIDS virus ENV protein expressed from a recombinant vaccinia virus. Biotechnology 1986; 4: 790-795.

82. Kilbourne ED. Influenza. In Wyngaarden JB, Smith LH eds. Cecil textbook of medicine. Philadelphia: W.B. Saunders Compnay, 1982: 1631-1635.

83. Klarman H, Guzick D. Economics of influenza. In Selby P ed. Influenza: virus, vaccine and strategy. New York: Academic Press, 1976: 255-270.

84. Klausner A. Controlled release delivery becoming key for biotech drugs. Biotechnology 1986; 49: 755-756.

85. Kleid DG. Using genetically engineered bacteria for vaccine production. Annals of the New York Academy of Sciences 1983; 413: 23-29.

86. Kohler G, Milstein C. Continuous cultures of fused cells secreting antibody of predefined specificity. Nature 1975; 256: 495-497.

87. Koplan JP. Benefits, risks, and costs of immunization programs (Manuscript). Atlanta, Georgia: Centers for Disease Control, 1984.

88. Koplan JP, Kane MA. Assessment of preventive health technology, the case of hepatitis B vaccine. Journal of Health Care Technology 1986; 2: 217-224.

89. Koplan J, Preblud S. A benefit-cost analysis of mumps vaccine. American Journal of Diseases of Children 1982; 136: 362-364.

90. Koplan J, Schoenbaum S, Weinstein M, Fraser D. Pertussis vaccine: an analysis of benefits, risks and costs. New England Journal of Medicine 1979; 300: 906-911.

91. Koplan JP, White CC. An update on the benefits and costs of measles and rubella immunization. In Gruenberg EM, Lewis C, Gadston S eds. Proceedings of the Conference of Two Agents that Endanger the Brain: Measles and Rubella. Baltimore, 1984.

92. Lafrenniere R, Rosenberg SA. Successful immunotherapy of murine experimental hepatic metastases with lymphokine activated killer cells and recombinant interleukin-2. Cancer Research 1985; 45: 3735-3741.

93. Lerner RA. Synthetic vaccines. Scientific American 1982; 251: 48-56.

94. Lerner RA, Green N, Alexander H, Liu F-T, Sutcliffe JG, Shinnick TM. Chemically synthesized peptides predicted from the nucleotide sequence of the hepatitis B virus genome elicit antibodies reactive with the native envelope protein of Dane particles. Proceedings of the National Academy of Sciences USA 1981; 78: 3403-3407.

95. Liew FY. New aspects of vaccine development. Clinical and Experimental Immunology 1985; 62: 225-241.

96. McAleer WJ, Buynak EB, Maigretter RZ, Wampler DE, Miller WJ, Hilleman MR. Human hepatitis B vaccine from recombinant yeast. Nature 1984; 307: 178-180.

97. McLean AA, Hilleman MR, McAleer WJ, Buynak EB. Summary of worldwide clinical experience with H-B-Vax (B,MSD). Journal of Infection 1983; 7: 95-104.

98. Massachusetts Public Health Department. Report on the measles, mumps, and rubella immunization programs. February 1979: 1-13.

99. Massachusetts Public Health Department. Report on the measles, mumps, and rubella immunization programs. March 1980: 1-13.

100. Maynard JE. Hepatitis B vaccine: strategies for utilization. In: Maupas P, Guesry P eds. Hepatitis B vaccine. INSERM symposium 18. New York: Elsevier, 1981: 13-19.

101. Mitchison NA. Rational design of vaccines. Nature 1984; 308: 112.

102. Mizel SB ed. Lymphokines in antibody and cytotoxic responses. New York: Academic Press, 1982.

103. Morein B. Iscom a new structure for antigenic presentation of membrane proteins. Vaccine 1985; 3: 155.

104. Moriarty AM, Hoyer BH, Shih JW, et al. Expression of the hepatitis B virus surface antigen gene in cell culture by using a simian virus 40 vector. National Academy of Sciences USA 1981; 78:2606-2610.

105. Mortimer IA. Pertussis. In Evans AS, Feldman HA, Bacterial infections of humans. New York: Plenum, 1982: 393-402.

106. Mule JJ, Shu S, Schwartz SL, Rosenberg SA. Adoptive immunotherapy of established pulmonary metastases with LAK cells and recombinant interleukin-2. Science 1984; 225: 1487-1489.

107. Mulley A, Silverstein, Dienstag J. Indications for use of hepatitis B vaccine, based on cost-effectiveness analysis. New England Journal of Medicine 1982; 307: 644-652.

108. National Institute of Allergy and Infectious Diseases. Status of vaccines targeted for accelerated development. Presented at Congressional Hearings on Biotechnology: Vaccine Development. Washington, DC: US Government Printing Office, 1985.

109. National Institute of Allergy and Infectious Diseases. Program for accelerated development of new vaccines: 1985 progress report. Washington, DC: US Government Printing Office, 1985.

110. Nisonoff A, Lamoyi E. Implications of the presence of an internal image of the antigen in anti-idiotypic antibodies: possible application to vaccine production. Clinical Immunology and Immunopathology 1981; 21: 397-406.

111. Norden CW. Haemophilus influenzae type b. In Evans AS, Feldman HA

eds. Bacterial infections of humans. New York: Plenum, 1981: 259-273.

112. Nowinski RC, Tam MR, Goldstein LC, Strong L, Kuo CC, Corey L, Stamm WE, Hansfield HH, Knapp JS, Holmes KK. Monoclonal antibodies for diagnosis of infectious diseases in humans. Science 1983; 219: 637-644.

113. Obrist R. Monoclonal antibodies as drug carriers in oncology. TIPS, 1983.

114. Ockner RK. Acute viral hepatitis. In Wyngaarden JB, Smith LH eds. Cecil textbook of medicine. Philadelphia: W.B. Saunders Compnay, 1982: 778-785.

115. Office of Technology Assessment. Blood policy & technology. Washington, DC: US Government Printing Office, 1985.

116. Office of Technology Assessment. Commercial biotechnology: an international analysis. Washington, DC: US Government Printing Office, 1984.

117. Office of Technology Assessment. Compensation for vaccine-related injuries. A technical memorandum. Washington, DC: US Government Printing Office, 1980.

118. Office of Technology Assessment. Cost-effectiveness analysis of influenza vaccine. Washington DC: US Government Printing Office, 1981.

119. Office of Technology Assessment. Impacts of applied genetics. Washington, DC: US Government Printing Office, 1981.

120. Office of Technology Assessment. The implications of cost-effectiveness analysis of medical technology. Washington, DC: US Government Printing Office, 1980.

121. Office of Technology Assessment. A review of selected federal vaccine and immunization policies. Washington, DC: US Government Printing Office, 1979.

122. Office of Technology Assessment. Update of federal activities regarding the use of pneumococcal vaccine. Washington, DC: US Government Printing Office, 1984.

123. Oldham RK. Biological response modifiers program. Journal of Biological Response Modifiers 1982; 1: 81-100.

124. Oldham RK. Biological response modifiers. Journal of the National Cancer Institute 1983; 70: 789-796.

125. Panicali D, Paoletti E. Construction of poxviruses as cloning vectors: insertion of the thymidine kinase gene of herpes simplex virus into the DNA of infectious vaccinia virus. Proceedings of the National Academy of Sciences of the United States of America 1982; 79: 4927-4931.

126. Pantell RH, Stewart TJ. The pneumococcal vaccine: immunization at a crossroad. Journal of the American Medical Association 1979; 241: 2272-2277.

127. Patrick K, Woolley FR. A cost-benefit analysis of immunization for pneumococcal pneumonia. Journal of the American Medical Association 1981; 245: 473-477.

128. Pennica D, Nedwin GE, Hayflich JS, Seeburg PH, Derynch R, Pallodino MA, Kohr WJ, Aggrawal BD, Goedell DV. Human tumor necrosis factor: precursor, structure, expression and homology to lymphotoxin. Nature 1984; 312: 724-728.

129. Perkins FT. Vaccination against communicable diseases. Symposia Series in Immunological Standardization 1973; 22: 1-407.

130. Pertola H, Kayhty H, Sivonen A, Makela PH. Haemophilus influenzae type by capsular polysaccharide vaccine in children: a double-bline field study of 100,000 vaccinees 3 months to 5 years of age in Finland. Pediatrics 1977; 60: 730-737.

131. Pertola H, Kayhty H, Virtanen M, Makela H. Prevention of Haemophilus influenzae type b bacteremic infections with the capsular polysaccharide vaccine. New England Journal of Medicine 1984; 310: 1561-1566.

132. Pinsky CM. Monoclonal Antibodies: progress is slow but sure. The New England Journal of Medicine, 1986; 315: 704-705.

133. Posey LM. Monoclonal antibodies have potential for diagnosis and treatment of disease. Clinical Pharmacology 1983; 2: 3.

134. Post LE, Roizman B. A generalized technique for the deletion of specific genes from large genomes: alpha gene 22 of herpes simplex virus 1 is not essential for growth. Cell 1981; 35: 227-232.

135. Prentis S. Biotechnology: a new industrial revolution. New York: George Braziller, inc., 1984.

136. Ratner L, Haseltine W, Patarca R, et al. Complete nucleotide sequence of the AIDS virus, HTLV-III. Nature 1985; 313: 277-284.

137. Reerink-Brongers EE, Reesink HW, Brummelhuis HGJ, et al. Preparation and evaluation of heat-inactivated HBsAg as a vaccine against hepatitis B. In Szmuness W, Alter HJ, Maynard JE eds. Viral Hepatitis: 1981 International Symposium. Philadelphia: Franklin Institute Press, 1982: 437-450.

138. Ritz J, Bast RC, Takvorian T, and Sallan SE. Clinical applications of monoclonal antibodies in acute leukemia. Annals of the New York Academy of Sciences 1984; 428: 308-318.

139. Rosen FS. The acquired immunodeficiency syndrome (AIDS). Journal of Clinical Investigation 1985; 75: 1-3.

140. Rosenberg SA, Lotze MT, Muul LM. A progress report on the treatment of 157 patients with advanced cancer using lymphokine-activating killer cells and interleukin-2 or high dose interleukin-2 alone. New England Journal of Medicine 1984; 44: 1946-1953.

141. Ruitenberg EJ. Vaccins. In: Toekomstverkenningen. Jaarboek Gezondheidsraad 1986. The Hague, The Netherlands: 59-70.

142. Schellekens H. Interferon, ontdekking, werking, toepassing. The Netherlands. Het Spectrum, 1982.

143. Schersten T. Home diagnostic tests. International Journal of Technology Assessment in Health Care 1985; 1: 441-442.

144. Schoenbaum S, Bartoshesky L, Crampton K. Benefit-cost analysis of rubella vaccination policy. New England Journal of Medicine 1976; 294: 306-310.

145. Schoenbaum S, McNeil B, Kavet J. The swine-flu decision. New England Journal of Medicine 1976; 295: 759-765.

146. Scott GM, Tyrell DAJ. Interferon: therapeutic fact or fiction for the 80s. British Medical Journal 1970; 28: 1558-1562.

147. Sela M. From antigens to synthetic vaccines. Biopolymers 1983; 22: 415-424.

148. Sigerist H. Man and medicine. Ciollege Park, Maryland: McGrath Publishing Company, 1970.

149. Skelly J, Howard CR, Zuckerman AJ. Hepatitis polypeptide vaccine preparation in micelle form. Nature 1981; 290: 51-54.

150. Smith GL, Mackett M, Moss B. Infectious vaccinia virus recombinants that express hepatitis B virus surface antigen. Nature 1983; 302: 490-495.

151. Smith, GL, Moss B, Uses of vaccinia virus as a vector for the production of live recombinant vaccines. Bio Essays 198 ; 1: 120-124.

152. Smith J, Pollard R. Vaccination against influenza: a five year study in the Post Office. Journal of Hygiene 1979; 83: 157-170.

153. Solnick D. Construction of an adenovirus SV40 recombinant producing T antigen from an adenovirus late promoter. Cell 1981; 24: 135-143.

154. Spaete RR, Frenkel N. The herpes simplex virus amplicon: a new eukaryotic defective cloning amplifying vector. Cell 1982; 30: 295-304.

155. Stevens CE, Taylor PE, Tong MJ, Toy PT, Vyas GN. Hepatitis B vaccine: an overview. Viral Hepatitis and Liver Disease 1984; 5: 275-291.

156. Stuart-Harris C. The present status of live influenza virus vaccine. Journal of Infectious Disease 1980; 142: 784-793.

157. Sugarman BJ, Aggarwal BB, Hass PE, Figari IS, Palladino MA, Shepard HM. Recombinant human tumor necrosis factor: effects on proliferation of normal and transformed cells in vitro. Science 1985; 230: 943-945.

158. Swartz MN. Bacterial meningitis. In Wyngaarden JB, Smith LH eds. Cecil textbook of medicine. Philadelphia: W.B. Saunders Compnay, 1982: 1473-1496.

159. Taverne JM, Dockrell J, Playfair JHL. Endotoxin-induced serum factor killed malarial parasites in vitro. Infectious Immunity 1981; 33: 83-89.

160. Valenzuela P, Medina A, Rutter WJ, et al. Synthesis and assembly

of hepatitis B virus surface antigen particles in yeast. Nature 1982; 298: 347-350.

161. Weis JH, Enquist LW, Salstrom JS, Watson RJ. An immunologically active chimaeric protein containing herpes simplex virus type 1 glycoprotein D. Nature 1983; 302: 72-74.

162. Weisbrod BA, Huston JH. Benefits and costs of human vaccines in developed countries: an evaluative survey. Madison, Wisconsin: Center for Health Economy and Law, University of Wisconsin-Madison, Discussion Paper #210, December 1983.

163. Weissman I. Approaches to understanding the pathogenic mechanisms in AIDS. Background paper. Washington, DC: Committee on a National Strategy for AIDS.

164. Wiedermann G, Ambrosch F. Costs and benefits of measles and mumps immunization in Austria. Bulletin of the World Health Organization 1979; 67: 625-629.

165. Willems J, Sanders C, Riddiough M, Bell J. Cost effectiveness of vaccination against pneumococcal pneumonia. New England Journal of Medicine 1980; 303: 553-559.

166. Winther MD, Dougan G. The impact of new technologies on vaccine development. Biotechnology and Genetic Engineering Reviews 1984; 2: 1-39.

167. Witte J, Axnick N. The benefits from 10 years of measles immunization in the United States. Public Health Reports 1975; 90: 205-207.

168. Wood IW, Capon DJ, Simonsen CC, Eaton DL, Gitschier J, Keyt B, et al. Expression of active human factor VIII from recombinant DNA clones. Nature 1984; 312: 330-337.

169. World Health Organization. Health research strategy for health for all 2000. Geneva, 1986.

170. World Health Organization. Hepatitis B vaccines prepared from yeast by recombinant DNA techniques, memorandum from a WHO meeting. Bulletin of the World Health Organization 1985; 63: 57-61.

171. World Health Organization. Immune responses to viral antigens in man and their relevance to vaccine development, memorandum from

a WHO meeting. Bulletin of the World Health Organization 1983; 61: 935-940.

172. World Health Organization. New approaches to vaccine development: memorandum from a WHO meeting. Bulletin of the World Health Organization 1985; 3: 479-484.

173. Zomerdijk JC. Diagnostic applications of monoclonal antibodies. A report issued to the Steering Committee on Future Health Scenarios. The Hague: CIVI, 1986.

174. Zuckerman AJ. Developing synthetic vaccines. Nature 1982; 295: 98-99.

175. Zuckerman AJ, Sun TT, Linsell A, Stjernward J. Prevention of primary liver cancer. Report on a meeting of a WHO Scientific Group. Lancet 1983; 1: 463-365.

www.ingramcontent.com/pod-product-compliance
Lightning Source LLC
Chambersburg PA
CBHW071926130926
51338CB00020B/42
* 9 7 8 0 8 9 8 3 8 4 1 2 3 *